THE

EVERYTHING®

GUIDE TO INTERMITTENT FASTING

Dear Reader,

If you would have told me ten years ago that purposefully skipping meals could balance my hormone levels, help me lose weight, boost my energy, reduce inflammation, and improve my brain health, I would have told you that you were crazy. Well, I might have been a little nicer about it, but I definitely would have thought you were crazy.

At the time, I was in my last year of my undergraduate program in nutrition and I was a firm believer that the key to health and maintaining a healthy weight was small, frequent meals throughout the day.

I actually stumbled upon intermittent fasting by accident, although at the time I didn't even know what it was. I got so busy with work and life that I just found myself skipping breakfast and forgetting to eat sometimes. Although I wasn't doing it on purpose, one day I realized that I felt better. I was sleeping better, I dropped a few excess pounds without trying to, and my anxiety levels went down. I also stopped obsessing about food—a problem I had dealt with throughout most of my time in college. I decided to dive in a little further, and that's when a whole new world opened up for me. When I started immersing myself into intermittent fasting, functional nutrition, and ancestral health, it just all made sense. Eat like our ancestors used to? Keep the body guessing? Sign me up for that.

It may seem counterintuitive that you could experience all of these health benefits by skipping meals, but stick with me. If you take the time to learn about intermittent fasting and how it affects your body and then, more importantly, take the time to try it for yourself, you may discover that getting back to basics has been the answer all along.

Lindsay Boyers, CHNC

Welcome to the EVERYTHING® Series!

These handy, accessible books give you all you need to tackle a difficult project, gain a new hobby, comprehend a fascinating topic, prepare for an exam, or even brush up on something you learned back in school but have since forgotten.

You can choose to read an Everything® book from cover to cover or just pick out the information you want from our four useful boxes: e-questions, e-facts, e-alerts, and e-ssentials.

We give you everything you need to know on the subject, but throw in a lot of fun stuff along the way too.

We now have more than 400 Everything® books in print, spanning such wide-ranging categories as weddings, pregnancy, cooking, music instruction, foreign language, crafts, pets, New Age, and so much more. When you're done reading them all, you can finally say you know Everything®!

QUESTION

Answers to common questions

FACT

Important snippets of information

ALERT

Urgent warnings

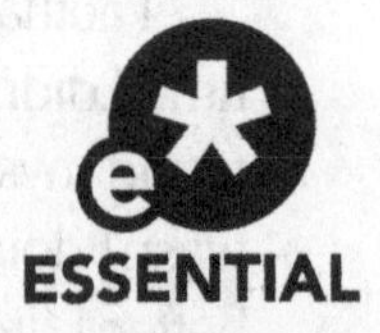

ESSENTIAL

Quick handy tips

PUBLISHER Karen Cooper

MANAGING EDITOR Lisa Laing

COPY CHIEF Casey Ebert

ASSOCIATE PRODUCTION EDITOR Jo-Anne Duhamel

ACQUISITIONS EDITOR Eileen Mullan

DEVELOPMENT EDITOR Sarah Doughty

EVERYTHING® SERIES COVER DESIGNER Erin Alexander

THE EVERYTHING® GUIDE TO INTERMITTENT FASTING

Features 5:2, 16/8, and Weekly 24-Hour Fast Plans

Lindsay Boyers, CHNC

Adams Media
New York London Toronto Sydney New Delhi

To JWM. Thank you for changing my world.

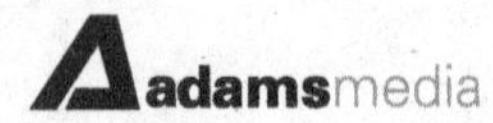

Adams Media
An Imprint of Simon & Schuster, Inc.
57 Littlefield Street
Avon, Massachusetts 02322

First Adams Media trade paperback edition December 2018

Manufactured in the United States of America

4 2025

Library of Congress Cataloging-in-Publication Data
Boyers, Lindsay, author.
The everything® guide to intermittent fasting / Lindsay Boyers, CHNC.
Avon, Massachusetts: Adams Media, 2018.
Series: Everything®.
Includes index.
LCCN 2018031903 (print) | LCCN 2018043928 (ebook) | ISBN 9781507208410 (pb) | ISBN 9781507208427 (ebook)
Subjects: LCSH: Fasting. | Diet. | Nutrition.
Classification: LCC RM226 (ebook) | LCC RM226 .B69 2018 (print) | DDC 613.2/5--dc23
LC record available at https://urldefense.proofpoint.com/v2/url?u=https-3A__lccn.loc.gov_2018031903&d=DwIFAg&c=jGUuvAdBXp_VqQ6t0yah2g&r=eLFfdQgpHVW0iSAzG8F-WtSjrFvCD9jGMJBHtzyExXhmHvwB7sjMCnFuKz95Uyqa&m=gktMXaWKOhv5EV4-IWStDlsWxMQShj26v6zcsex1YDs&s=TxO0c_tuEj09WrsL8qXg6PKFRHxqPD0dBNVBX4bJ_7o&e=

ISBN 978-1-5072-0841-0
ISBN 978-1-5072-0842-7 (ebook)

Always follow safety and commonsense cooking protocols while using kitchen utensils, operating ovens and stoves, and handling uncooked food. If children are assisting in the preparation of any recipe, they should always be supervised by an adult.

Contains material adapted from the following titles published by Adams Media, an Imprint of Simon & Schuster, Inc.: *The Everything® Paleolithic Diet Slow Cooker Cookbook* by Emily Dionne, MS, RD, LDN, CSSD, ACSM-HFS, copyright © 2013, ISBN 978-1-4405-5536-7; *The Everything® Paleolithic Diet Book* by Jodie Cohen and Gilaad Cohen, copyright © 2011, ISBN 978-1-4405-1206-3; *The Everything® Low-FODMAP Diet Cookbook* by Colleen Francioli, CNC, copyright © 2016, ISBN 978-1-4405-9529-5; *The Everything® Mediterranean Cookbook* by Dawn Altomari-Rathjen, LPN, BPS, and Jennifer M. Bendelius, MS, RD, copyright © 2003, ISBN 978-1-58062-869-3; *The Everything® Vegetarian Cookbook* by Jay Weinstein, copyright © 2002, ISBN 978-1-58062-640-8; *The Everything® Eating Clean Cookbook* by Britt Brandon, CFNS, CPT, copyright © 2012, ISBN 978-1-4405-2999-3; *The Everything® Candida Diet Book* by Jeffrey McCombs, DC, copyright © 2014, ISBN 978-1-4405-7523-5; *The Everything® Healthy Green Drinks Book* by Britt Brandon, copyright © 2014, ISBN 978-1-4405-7694-2; *The Everything® Thyroid Diet Book* by Clara Schneider, MS, RD, RN, CDE, LDN, copyright © 2011, ISBN 978-1-4405-1097-7; *The Everything® Vegan Cookbook* by Jolinda Hackett with Lorena Novak Bull, RD, copyright © 2010, ISBN 978-1-4405-0216-3; *The Everything® Guide to the Autoimmune Diet* by Dr. Jeffrey McCombs, DC, copyright © 2015, ISBN 978-1-4405-8732-0.

Contents

Introduction

HAVE YOU HEARD THAT intermittent fasting can help you lose weight? Are you looking to gain muscle and drop those extra pounds? If so, you're in the right place. Intermittent fasting can do both of those things...but that's not all it can do. The benefits of intermittent fasting extend far beyond weight loss—from immune-system enhancement to inflammation prevention. That's right: skipping meals can improve your total health!

Strategically skipping meals also balances your blood sugar and insulin levels, which in turn can improve mental clarity, reduce your risk of type 2 diabetes, heart disease, and fat gain, and protect you from developing neurodegenerative diseases like dementia and Alzheimer's disease. And if you're looking to delay the effects of aging, intermittent fasting can help there too. Intermittent fasting places temporary stress on your cells; over time, as your body acclimates to dealing with stress, it becomes better at delaying aging processes by more effectively repairing physical injuries, fighting off disease, and gaining muscle mass.

Of course, like anything nutrition- and diet-related, it's important to learn the basics and your specific body's needs, and also to experiment with which plan is right for you. In *The Everything® Guide to Intermittent Fasting*, you'll discover everything you need to be successful, no matter your reasons for fasting. You'll learn more about each of the following popular fasting methods:

- 16/8—Fast for sixteen hours and eat within the remaining eight hours eat day.
- Eat Stop Eat—Eat regularly for five days each week and fast for the remaining two days.
- 5:2—Eat regularly for five days each week and eat two meals each day for the remaining two days.
- Alternate day—Alternate between eating regularly one day and eating two meals the next.

Each method comes with unique advantages: the 16/8 method is more scheduled and focused on the day-to-day process, while the Eat Stop Eat, 5:2, and alternate day methods are more flexible and focused on the week as a whole. Are you unsure of which schedule would be best? In these chapters, you'll learn exactly which method is right for you.

Chapters 7–11 are full of 150 delicious, healthy recipes. From Tomato Spinach Frittata Muffins to South American Chili, these easy-to-make dishes will keep you full no matter which way you choose to fast. While many of the recipes are heartier so you are able to fit all of your nutritional needs into your fasting schedule with ease, some recipes are less than 500 calories (marked by an * symbol), for those feeding windows when you are in the mood for something a bit lighter or for a snack to tide you over in between larger meals. In addition to these recipes, you'll find detailed two-week meal plans for each fasting type.

With *The Everything® Guide to Intermittent Fasting*, you'll be on your way to a healthier, happier you in no time!

CHAPTER 1

The Basics of Intermittent Fasting

Although it may seem like you're hearing a lot more about it recently, intermittent fasting is not a new concept. In fact, fasts have been an important part of history and religion for centuries. Many people are starting to catch on to the health benefits of fasting, from a boost in energy to weight loss and increased mental clarity. In this chapter, you'll learn what exactly intermittent fasting is and the basic science underlying it. You'll discover the difference between a "fed" state and a "fasted" state (the metabolic states upon which intermittent fasting is built). You'll also be given a brief overview of the history of intermittent fasting and how various religions incorporate fasting into their spiritual practices.

What Is Intermittent Fasting?

Intermittent fasting isn't a specific diet plan. It's a general term that describes an eating pattern in which you alternate between eating and fasting (purposefully going without food for a set period of time). To fully understand intermittent fasting, it's helpful to know the difference between a "fed" state and a "fasted" state—the two phases of the digestive system.

Fed versus Fasted States

A fed state—also called the absorptive state—happens right after a meal or a snack, when your body is digesting the food and absorbing its nutrients. As soon as you even think about, see, or smell food, and your mouth starts to water, digestion begins. It continues until the broken-down components of your food are transported into your blood, where they travel to the liver, fatty (or adipose) tissue, and muscles.

When the broken-down components of food first enter your blood, it causes your blood glucose levels to rise, which then stimulates the beta cells (the specialized cells in your pancreas that produce, store, and release insulin) to release insulin into the blood. The released insulin then attaches to the glucose in your blood and carries it to the cells, where it's used for energy, or carries it to the liver and muscles, where it's converted to glycogen and stored for later use.

In the fed state, which typically lasts for four hours, insulin is elevated, which prompts your body to store any excess calories in the fat cells. While insulin is elevated, your body also stops burning fat and turns instead to glucose (from the food you just ingested) for energy.

Once the fed state ends, your body enters the fasted, or postabsorptive, state. This state begins after the food has been digested, absorbed, and properly stored. When you're in the fasted state, approximately four hours after you eat, your body relies on stored glycogen for energy. Glucose levels in the blood drop as the cells begin to use the sugar, and in response to this decrease in glucose, insulin levels drop as well. Because your body likes to maintain blood glucose levels between 70 and 99 milligrams per deciliter, this drop in glucose in the blood triggers the alpha cells of the pancreas to release a hormone called glucagon. Glucagon travels to the liver, where it breaks glycogen down into glucose. Once glucose is formed, it's released by the liver and travels to your brain and tissues.

In this fasted state, insulin and glucose levels are low, while glucagon and growth-hormone levels are high. After the glucose that comes from the stored glycogen is used up, the body turns to stored fat in your fat cells for energy, burning up the fat in the process.

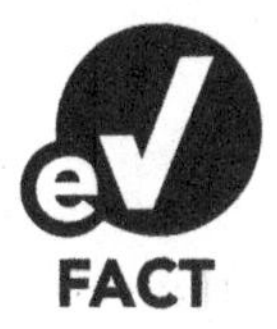

Your body more effectively burns stored fat when you're in a fasted state. When you're in a fed state, your body stores more fat. If you're eating every two to three hours each day, your body never enters a fasted state, since the fed state lasts for approximately four hours.

The Mechanisms of Starvation

The fed state and fasted state are two of the main metabolic states of the body, but there's also a third metabolic state: starvation. When the body is deprived of nutrients for an extended period of time, it goes into "starvation mode," or adaptive thermogenesis. Many people think that the starvation mode will kick in after only a few hours of eating (this is where the advice to eat five to six small meals throughout the day came from), but it doesn't work like that. Starvation mode only kicks in when the glucose that's stored in the liver (technically called glycogen) is depleted. The glycogen in your liver can last for twelve to twenty-four hours, on average, although if you're doing strenuous exercise or endurance training, it can zap up glycogen more quickly than that.

Your body's only job is survival, so its top priority at all times is to provide enough glucose to fuel your brain. The second priority is to conserve amino acids to make new proteins, instead of breaking down and using them for energy. Because of this, when you enter starvation mode and your body doesn't have excess glucose or glycogen to use for your brain's needs, it will turn to ketones, which are organic compounds created from fatty acids. In order to create these ketones, your body will break down fatty acids and triglycerides from your fat stores. Since your brain and the rest of your body can use ketones for energy instead of glucose, this prevents the breakdown of proteins and saves you from losing muscle density.

The ketogenic diet, a high-fat, very low-carbohydrate diet, is based on the physiology of the starvation metabolic state. Keep in mind that although this state is biologically classified as starvation, you're not technically starving. When following a proper ketogenic diet, you're providing your body with the nutrients it needs to continue creating the ketone bodies that will serve as its main fuel source.

The primary goal of intermittent fasting is to limit the amount of time your body spends in a fed state and to extend the length of time your body is in a fasted state. Aside from all of the health benefits that come with it, two of the major pros to intermittent fasting are that you get to choose both your fasting and feeding windows and you get to choose what diet works best for you.

A History of Fasting

When it comes to the history of civilization, easy, regular access to food is actually a fairly new concept. Before the Industrial Revolution, people had to rely solely on the land to get food. They couldn't simply take a ride to their nearest grocery store anytime they needed to fill their stomachs. Ancient civilizations (and some civilizations around the world today) hunted and gathered as much as they could, but food wasn't always a guarantee. Sometimes the hunters and gatherers would come back with a fresh kill and a load of fresh fruit and berries; other days, especially in times of scarcity like the winter months, they would come back empty-handed. Although they weren't doing it intentionally, they were essentially fasting on these days. Depending on the time of the year and the skill of the hunters and gatherers, these fasts could last days, weeks, or even months.

Aside from this unintentional fasting, some ancient civilizations caught on to the benefits of fasting well before modern research. The ancient Greeks believed that fasting could improve your cognitive abilities and concentration. Benjamin Franklin, one of America's founding fathers and the claimed inventor of the lightning rod and bifocal glasses, wrote, "The best of all medicines is resting and fasting."

Spiritual Fasting

Fasting has also been—and remains—an important part of various religions and spiritual practices around the world. When used for religious purposes, fasting is often described as a cleansing or a purification process, but the basic concept is still the same: abstain from eating for a set period of time.

Unlike medical fasting, which is used as a treatment for illness, spiritual fasting is seen as an important catalyst to whole-body wellness, and a wide variety of religions share the belief that fasting has the power to heal. In Buddhism, fasting is a way to practice restraint from acting on human desires, a restraint that Buddhist monks believe is a piece of the puzzle to achieving nirvana. Many Buddhists fast daily, eating food in the morning but abstaining for the rest of the day, until it is time to eat the next morning. In addition to this, Buddhists often embark on a water-only fast for days or weeks.

In Christianity, fasting is a way to cleanse the soul so that the body is pure and so that a connection with God can be made. One of the most popular times that Christians fast is called Lent, the forty-day period between Ash Wednesday and Easter. In earlier days, those observing Lent gave up food or drink; in more modern times, Christians might still abstain from food or drink but often choose instead to go without a specific thing. This practice is meant to be an acknowledgment of the forty days that Jesus Christ spent in the desert, forced to fast.

In Hinduism, it's believed that denying the physical needs of the body by fasting helps increase spirituality. Although fasting is a regular part of the Hindu religion and is done often, one of the most popular observed fasts is during Maha Shivaratri, or the "Great Night of Shiva." During Maha Shivaratri, devotees fast, take part in ritual baths, visit a temple where they pray, and practice the virtues of honesty, forgiveness, and self-discipline.

In Judaism, there are several reasons to fast, including asking for God's mercy, marking important life events, showing gratitude to God, or mourning; however, if you are doing an individual fast, it is custom to keep the fast private.

In Mormonism, there's a tradition called Fast Sunday, in which followers abstain from two meals (for a period of twenty-four hours) on the first Sunday of every month. During this fast, members share personal stories with their church community in an extra effort to cleanse and purify. They also donate the equivalent cost of those two meals to the church to provide assistance to the needy—a practice known as a fast offering.

Perhaps the most well-known religious fast, Ramadan, is a part of the Muslim religion. During Ramadan, Muslims not only abstain from food and drink from dusk to dawn, but they also avoid smoking, sexual relations, and any other activities that may be viewed as sinful. The period of fasting—and the mild dehydration that occurs from lack of fluids—is believed to cleanse the soul of harmful impurities so that the heart can be redirected to spirituality and away from earthly desires.

Of course, these are just a few of the religions that incorporate fasting into their worship. Other religions that incorporate fasting include Baha'i, Jainism, Sikhism, Taoism, Anglicanism, Methodism, Pentecostalism, Lutheranism, and Catholicism.

Medical Fasting

Hippocrates, who's been given the nickname "The Father of Medicine," introduced fasting as a medical therapy for some of his sick patients as far back as the fifth century B.C.E. One of Hippocrates's famous quotes states, "To eat when you are sick is to feed your illness." He believed that fasting allowed the body to focus on healing itself, and that forcing food in a diseased state could actually be detrimental to a person's health because instead of giving the necessary energy to healing, your body would use all of its available energy on digestion. On the other hand, if sick patients abstained from food, digestive processes would shut down and the body would prioritize natural healing.

In addition to avoiding food, medical fasts, which were popular around 400 B.C.E., often involved excessive exercise and enemas. The belief was that by boosting elimination—through sweat and the removal of bodily waste—when digestion was shut down, any excess toxins would be removed from the body, allowing the body to heal to a greater degree.

Some of these medical fasts allowed only water and calorie-free tea for up to one month, while others allowed patients to consume 200–500 calories per day. These calories typically came from bread, broths, juices, and milk. The specific details of the fast depended on the person's condition.

All medical fasts that require patients to abstain completely from food for up to one month should be monitored by a physician. While intermittent fasting is perfectly safe for most people, you should never attempt to go more than twenty-four hours without eating unless you have supervision or approval from your healthcare provider.

However, it wasn't until the 1900s that fasting started appearing in scientific journals as an effective medical therapy for obesity and other illnesses; even then, the benefits didn't fully catch on until more recently.

The Science Behind the Fast

Like any nutritional concept that quickly takes over health and diet communities, intermittent fasting has been accused of being a fad, but the science behind the benefits of fasting is already clear—and growing. There are several theories as to why intermittent fasting works so well, but the most frequently studied—and most proven—benefit has to do with stress.

The word *stress* has been vilified time and time again, but some stress is actually beneficial to your body. For example, exercise is technically a stress to the body (to the muscles and the cardiovascular system, specifically), but this particular stress ultimately makes the body stronger, as long as you incorporate the right amount of recovery time into your exercise routine.

According to Mark Mattson, who is the senior investigator for the National Institute on Aging, intermittent fasting stresses the body in the same way exercise does. When you deny the body food for a set period of time, it puts the cells under mild stress. Over time cells adapt to this stress by learning how to cope with it better. When your body is better at dealing with stress, it has an increased ability to resist disease.

Good Stress versus Bad Stress

While some types of stress are good for the body, helping it to adapt and grow, other types of stress aren't. It's important to distinguish between "good" and "bad" stresses so that you can get a handle on the bad ones. When you're exposed to stress, a part of your brain called the amygdala recognizes that stress as a threat to your health. In response to this threat, the amygdala sends a message to another part of your brain, called the hypothalamus, to release corticotrophin-releasing hormone, or CRH. CRH then stimulates yet another part of your brain, called the pituitary gland, to release adrenocorticotropic hormone, or ACTH. The release of ACTH signals the adrenal glands to produce and release cortisol. The adrenal glands also release adrenaline, which elevates your blood pressure and increases your heart rate. The presence of cortisol helps maintain proper blood pressure and fluid balance, while temporarily shutting down some body functions, like digestion, to preserve energy. In this case, once the immediate threat goes away, cortisol levels drop back down and normal body functions are resumed.

Good stress, also referred to as eustress, is a mild stress that most people experience on a regular basis. Instead of being harmful to the body, eustress inspires you and propels you to reach a goal or a desired outcome, and it's generally associated with some type of happiness or excitement when that goal is achieved. Examples of eustress include training for an athletic event, working toward a deadline, or practicing for an upcoming performance. Research shows that eustress can actually improve your brain function. The defining characteristic of eustress is that it is short-lasting. Once the goal is met or the project is finished, eustress goes away and your cortisol levels drop back down and normalize, giving your body time to recover.

Bad stress, or what is otherwise known as distress, is chronic, unrelenting stress that hinders your productivity or gets in the way of your daily life. Instead of pushing you to achieve your goals, distress makes it harder to achieve them. Distress keeps your cortisol and adrenaline levels high, which can lead to weakened adrenal glands and problems with normal hormonal signaling. Some chronic health problems linked to distress include depression, heart disease, weight gain, and a greater susceptibility to illnesses like colds and flus. Examples of distress include toxic romantic relationships, constant work stress, and trauma or death in the family.

However, because everyone reacts differently to certain things and has a different perspective on life, the line between good and bad stress can become blurred. The best way to determine whether something is eustress or distress for you is to ask yourself a few questions. Does it make you feel challenged, yet motivated? If so, it's likely good stress. Does it make you feel overwhelmed, withdrawn, and tired? If so, it's probably bad stress.

Is Fasting Right for You?

Fasting is appropriate for most healthy people, but there are certain groups of people who shouldn't fast or who should speak to their healthcare team before starting a fast.

You should not fast if you:

- Are pregnant or breastfeeding
- Are under eighteen years of age
- Are severely underweight or malnourished

You should speak to your healthcare provider before fasting if you:

- Have diabetes (type 1 or type 2)
- Are taking any medications
- Have gout
- Have GERD (gastroesophageal reflux disease)
- Have cortisol dysregulation or are under severe stress
- Have a history of disordered eating

Even if you don't fall into any of these categories, listen carefully to your body to determine if fasting is right for you. If you're feeling low in energy or lightheaded upon standing, you may have to adjust your fasting window or check in with your doctor to make sure your body can regulate your blood sugar properly. Keep in mind that it can take a long time for your body to adjust to your new lifestyle. There is typically a three- to six-week transition period during which your body and your brain adapt to fasting. During this time, you may experience hunger, irritability, weakness, and even loss of libido. This is a normal response, but if symptoms are severe, work with your healthcare provider during these initial stages. If you feel great after the adjustment period, then it's a good sign that your body likes what you're doing. If you feel dizzy, lightheaded, or low on energy after this period, then you should stop fasting and speak with your healthcare provider.

Fasting and Diabetes

Fasting can be a challenge for those with diabetes because the body has a harder time regulating blood-glucose and insulin levels than it does in people who don't have diabetes. However, research shows that intermittent fasting may be beneficial in helping to return glucose levels to normal. The biggest concern when it comes to fasting and diabetes is hypoglycemia, or low blood sugar.

If you have diabetes, make sure that you have your doctor's approval and supervision before starting any type of fast. If your doctor approves intermittent fasting, familiarize yourself with the symptoms of low blood sugar and have a plan in place for treating your blood sugar levels if they get too low. If blood sugar levels exceed 300 milligrams per deciliter or drop below 70 milligrams per deciliter, stop the fast immediately and apply the proper treatment. Hypoglycemia is more likely to occur in those with type 1 diabetes than those with type 2 diabetes. Signs of hypoglycemia include:

- Fatigue
- Shakiness
- Hunger
- Irritability
- Anxiety
- Increased sweating
- Irregular heartbeat
- Pale skin

Severe hypoglycemia may cause:

- Confusion
- Blurred vision
- Abnormal behavior or mental confusion
- Loss of consciousness
- Seizure

If you experience any of these symptoms, seek medical attention.

Fasting and "Bad" Stress

The stress that fasting puts on the body can be categorized as eustress for most people. It's mild and it results in health benefits that can push you to keep going to achieve your ultimate goals. However, if you're under chronic distress already, you'll want to get that under control before you incorporate intermittent fasting into your routine. In the case of chronic stress, your body is continuously pumping out cortisol. When cortisol levels stay elevated for an extended period of time, it can lead to:

- Anxiety
- Depression
- Weight gain
- Headaches
- Problems with memory and concentration
- Difficulty sleeping
- Digestive issues
- Heart disease

Over time chronic stress also affects the function of your adrenal glands negatively and makes it harder for them to regulate hormones properly.

If you're already under a great deal of chronic stress, getting your cortisol levels under control and your adrenal glands working properly before beginning to fast is extremely important. You can reduce cortisol levels by meditating, avoiding coffee, getting enough sleep, following a clean, healthy diet for a period of time before incorporating fasting, and avoiding excessive exercise. Low-impact, meditative exercises like yoga can be helpful.

Yoga

In a study conducted by the Yoga Research Society and the Sidney Kimmel Medical College of Thomas Jefferson University, researchers found that cortisol levels dropped significantly after a fifty-minute yoga class that included popular yoga poses like the tree pose, plow pose, and locust pose. Researchers believe that this drop in cortisol is due in part to the activation of the relaxation response through the holding of poses and deep breathing.

This relaxation response shuts off the stress cascade, and as a result stress hormones are naturally reduced.

High cortisol levels are also common in those with depression. A study published in the *Indian Journal of Psychiatry* found that yoga may help shut off the stress response in the hypothalamus section of the brain, which can bring relief of symptoms to those with depression. In fact, the study found that yoga dropped cortisol levels better than antidepressants did.

Meditation

Research suggests that daily meditation doesn't just feel good in the moment: it can actually alter the brain's neural pathways, reducing anxiety and making you more resistant to stress and resilient. There's no right or wrong way to meditate, so don't let your preconceived notions about what meditation is supposed to be deter you from starting your own routine. If you're new to meditation, you can start by following along with some guided meditations. You can access thousands of meditation videos online to help get you started.

Deep Breathing

Meditation and deep breathing go hand in hand, but you can do some quick deep-breathing exercises on your own, too, whenever you feel stress building up—or even when you don't and you want to stay ahead of it.

When you're stressed, you tend to take quick, shallow breaths that come from your chest rather than your abdomen. When you breathe deeply from your abdomen instead, you take in more oxygen, which helps you feel less anxious, less short of breath, and more relaxed. Learning how to take deep breaths takes practice, but the following steps will make it easy for you to become a pro deep-breather in no time:

1. Sit up straight or lie on your back somewhere comfortable. Put one hand on your chest and the other on your abdomen.
2. Take a deep breath in through your nose. You should feel the hand on your abdomen rise, but the hand on your chest should move very little.

3. Exhale through your mouth, pushing out as much air as you can.
4. Repeat this process until you feel your body start to relax.

Journaling

Getting your thoughts and frustrations out on paper has a proven positive effect on stress levels. You can also use your journal to create daily gratitude lists. Writing down just three things you're grateful for every day will help you further reduce your stress by reminding you of the positive things in your life. They don't have to be big things. In fact, taking stock of the little things in your life will help you appreciate your day-to-day experiences even more. You can write down things like, "I'm grateful that I have a bed to sleep in," or, "I'm grateful for this cup of coffee." Try to choose different things every day and you'll see how much you really have to be thankful for—even things that you might not have paid much attention to before.

Journaling is also helpful for keeping track of your emotions and how these emotions affect your eating habits. Write down how you feel each day as well as what you're eating. When you look back at the pages, you'll be able to recognize how your emotions connect with food (the amount and types that you're eating) and you'll be able to focus on breaking negative behavior patterns that you might not have been aware of otherwise.

Music

You know that feeling when your favorite song comes on and you start to sing along and immediately feel better? There's science behind that. Research shows that regardless of what mood you're in, listening to music that you love can lower your cortisol levels. Although any music that you love can have a stress-lowering effect, classical music shows great results. Listening to classical music can lower stress hormones, decrease blood pressure, and slow down both your pulse and your heart rate.

In addition to the physical effects, music also diverts your attention. Instead of getting caught up in your thoughts or incessant mind chatter, music absorbs your attention and forces you to focus on something else. So, the next time you're feeling stressed, turn on some classical music or a song that you love. Lie down and listen or even dance it out.

Social Connectedness

Studies show that close human bonds are essential to both your physical and mental health and that social isolation can lead to increased levels of cortisol. Human touch actually stimulates your vagus nerve (one of the nerves that connects your brain to your body), relaxing your nervous system and shutting down your stress response. Touch also increases the release of oxytocin (a hormone linked to feelings of relaxation, trust, and mental stability)—sometimes referred to as the "love hormone"—and reduces the release of cortisol.

Face-to-face contact is best, so find as much time to connect with your loved ones as possible. Surround yourself with supportive people who want to see you succeed in your goals; avoid people who are combative or whom you don't get along with. Tense relationships can increase cortisol levels.

Getting Ready to Fast

With the exception of spontaneous fasting, most types of intermittent fasting require some preparation. One of the most important things you can do to prepare for your fast is to develop a plan. What type of intermittent fasting will you be doing? During which days and times will you fast? What is your official start date? It's helpful to write out a schedule for yourself and keep it where you can see it all the time. You can even set timers on your phone to go off when it's time to begin your fast and when it's time to start eating again. But you also don't have to jump in to a set fasting schedule right away: you can ease yourself in slowly to get the hang of it.

Easing Into Your Fast

If you're new to intermittent fasting or you're used to eating five or six small meals or constantly grazing throughout the day, it can be a big transition to jump right into fasting. You don't have to make a complete change overnight; in fact, you may be more successful if you slowly ease yourself into it.

Start by transitioning from five or six small meals throughout the day to three normal-sized, timed meals. You don't have to eat within a certain window of time yet, just get your body used to the habit and the structure of the three-meal schedule. This will also require you to eliminate snacking throughout the day. Snacking isn't forbidden when you're intermittent fasting, but it can be helpful to eliminate snacks during the beginning stages when you're adjusting. As your body gets used to fasting, you can incorporate snacks during the day, as long as you eat them during your feeding window.

Once you've gotten the hang of a three-meal schedule, choose one meal to skip and commit to skipping it each day for a couple of weeks. Don't spend too much time thinking about which meal to skip; you can switch meals later if it works better for you or your schedule. The point is to get your body used to going without food for an extended period of time. Sometimes the hardest part of fasting is training your mind to accept the thought of skipping meals, so this will get you used to that idea.

Once you've gotten the hang of skipping meals and you've chosen which eating plan you're going to follow, slowly work your way up to the ultimate fasting goal. For example, if you're going to follow the 16/8 method and you've decided that your eating window is going to fall between eleven a.m. and seven p.m., but you normally eat breakfast at seven thirty a.m., start by pushing breakfast back to eight thirty a.m. for a couple of days. Then when you're used to the later breakfast, push it back another hour, and then another hour in a few more days until your body is comfortable with waiting until eleven a.m. to eat. Gradually pushing back your eating times won't just help ease you into the fast mentally, it may also help prevent or decrease some of the initial physical symptoms that can occur during the beginning stages of intermittent fasting.

The next steps are to figure out what type of eating plan you're going to follow and to find some new and delicious recipes to incorporate into your plan. Fancy, intricate recipes are always tempting—and can be a great treat on the weekends—but in the initial stages of your new fasting plan, it will be easier to keep things simple. Choose recipes that are easy to prepare and made with easily accessible ingredients.

When you're just starting out with intermittent fasting, it's also helpful to scale back on your workout routine. In the very beginning stages of fasting, you may be low on energy and motivation. That's perfectly normal. Instead of engaging in any high-intensity exercises, keep your workouts light. Try yoga, brisk walking, or swimming. If you normally do higher-intensity training or a lot of strength training, it might feel counterintuitive to cut back, but you can resume your workout routine in a couple of weeks when your body has adjusted.

CHAPTER 2

What to Expect

As with any lifestyle change, intermittent fasting may be difficult at first. You may experience some irritability or a drop in energy. You may feel really hungry and have a hard time sticking to your plan. Or you might feel great right off the bat, experiencing positive results immediately and feeling energized and motivated by your new lifestyle. It depends on your body. However, there are some things that are likely to occur as you adjust to your new routine. When you know what to expect and you have some tools ready to cope with any challenges that may arise, your chances for long-term success are much greater.

How Your Mind Will Feel

There's a popular quote that says, "Your mind will quit a thousand times before your body will," and another quote that states, "Your body can stand almost anything. It's your mind you have to convince." The general message behind both of these powerful quotes is that often, when you give up, it's not because you've actually reached your physical limit, it's because you've reached your mental limit. In other words, your mind convinces you that your body can't physically handle a challenge, when it actually can.

The Negativity Bias

Your brain has a tendency to react more strongly to negative things than it does to positive things. This phenomenon is called the negativity bias—and it can be extremely powerful. The biological purpose of the negativity bias is to protect you from possible threats, but in modern times, threats like those faced by your ancestors are fewer and farther between. As a result, you don't need this negativity bias as often, because it's not as helpful as it once was. In fact, this bias makes it harder for you be present and calm, because you're always on alert and anticipating a negative event instead of appreciating the moment. The good news is that you can actually retrain your brain so that it doesn't revert to the negativity bias as easily.

The Power of Positive Thinking

Positive thinking and affirmations are not just New Age trends: they're powerful tools that can actually rewire the neurons in your brain—a concept known as neuroplasticity. When you regularly engage in positive thinking and repeat positive affirmations, it makes it easier for your brain to respond more positively to things rather than immediately resorting to its natural negativity bias. And the more you practice, the easier it becomes for your brain to think positively.

When you're starting out with intermittent fasting, your subconscious mind will resist the change and will do all it can to get you to resort back to your old routine. When you know this, it's easier to become aware of negative thought patterns and unconstructive self-talk. You may find yourself thinking things like, "This is way too hard," "I'm starving," or "A small snack outside of my fasting window won't hurt." These thoughts are all indications that your negativity bias is running the show. When your mind starts to tell you that it's too hard, recognize that it is this bias talking and respond by saying something like, "I'm stronger than my thoughts. I can and will meet my goals."

Neuroplasticity refers to the brain's ability to change and adapt to an environment. The brain goes through physiological changes from the day you're born to the end of your life. Neurogenesis is the formation of new brain cells. Like neuroplasticity, neurogenesis also happens throughout your life but only in certain areas of the brain.

In addition to regularly practicing positive affirmations and changing your negative self-talk, you can also shut your negativity bias down by focusing on the bigger picture. Figure out your main reasons for fasting. Is it to lose weight? Gain more mental clarity and energy? Balance your blood sugar levels? Keep your brain healthy? Whatever your reasons are, write them on a piece of paper or sticky notes and keep them somewhere you will see them frequently, like on the refrigerator. When you feel these negative thoughts start to creep in, read the notes and remember your main goals and why you started in the first place. This can help you see the bigger picture, which will get you through any little speed bumps along the way.

Once you get past the initial stages of intermittent fasting, it's likely that you'll notice some major changes. Not only will your negative self-talk and negativity bias diminish, but you'll also experience more mental clarity. Intermittent fasting tends to lift brain fog and make concentration easier. You may find that simple tasks become easier and that you're able to focus on your work more. You may also experience less "monkey mind"—intrusive, rapid thoughts that distract you from the task at hand and interfere with your productivity. You may notice your productivity and energy levels increasing. Your memory may feel sharper, and retaining new information may become easier than it was before. You may also notice a stabilization in your moods and emotions—even less anxiety and a more cheerful disposition.

How Your Body Will Feel

It's impossible to say exactly how your body will feel during the initial stages of intermittent fasting, since everyone is different and you may respond differently than someone else. However, there are a few things that commonly occur in most people when starting intermittent fasting. If you're used to eating five or six times per day, you may experience these effects to a greater degree than if you already eat three meals a day with minimal snacking.

As your body adjusts to intermittent fasting, it's normal to feel increased hunger and cravings. Often this is mental or emotional hunger rather than physical hunger. You may also experience headaches, low energy, and irritability. It's possible to feel a little dizzy, weak, or light-headed upon standing. The severity of these symptoms can vary based on several factors, including your previous eating habits, but they shouldn't be extremely intrusive, and they should diminish within a week or so.

FACT

If you are experiencing severe symptoms that don't go away or improve, discontinue your fast immediately and speak with your healthcare provider. It could be a sign of blood sugar problems that require medical supervision.

After the initial adjustment period, your blood sugar and insulin levels start to stabilize and you'll begin to reap the benefits of intermittent fasting. One of the first things you'll likely notice is increased energy. You may feel a sustained energy throughout the day, instead of feeling awake and productive in the morning but then being hit with that dreaded afternoon slump around two or three p.m., you'll feel constant energy. This is because your blood sugar isn't spiking and dropping like it does when you eat several meals over the course of the entire day.

You may also experience a decrease in inflammation, so any puffiness in your face, skin, hands, or feet may start to diminish. Chronic aches and pains that became a regular part of your day may reduce or go away completely. Then you might start to notice that you're dropping a few extra pounds, that you fall asleep easier, and that the quality of your sleep is better. You'll toss and turn less at night and as a result you'll wake up feeling refreshed and rested instead of groggy and disoriented. If you're exercising regularly, you might also find it easier to get through your workouts.

A good way to keep track of changes is to write down any symptoms you feel before starting your intermittent fasting plan. Try to dig deep and be really comprehensive, even listing things that you've dealt with for a long time or that you think have nothing to do with your eating habits. After you've been fasting for a couple of weeks, go back and rewrite your list and compare the two lists. Rewrite your list every couple of weeks after that. This can help you track improvements that you may not even be expecting, and it's likely that you'll be pleasantly surprised.

Staving Off Hunger

In the initial stages of intermittent fasting you're going to feel hungry—there's no way around that. Luckily, with an understanding of hunger cues and a few easy techniques, you can stave off both physical and mental hunger without breaking your fast.

The Psychology of Hunger

Hunger is tricky because, on one hand, there's true, physiological hunger; on the other hand, there's mental hunger. Put simply: physical hunger occurs when your stomach is empty. You may feel the physical emptiness in your stomach along with a weakness or a dip in energy. Psychological hunger is the result of a desire to eat out of habit or boredom or because of external cues. While you may do these things subconsciously, when you become aware of them, you can change how they affect you. Instead of mindlessly eating because you're at a social event or your significant other is hungry, pay attention to how you really feel. Are you truly hungry, or are you just tempted by one of these cues? If it's the latter, you can either change your environment or use one of a few helpful techniques provided in this chapter for curbing your hunger.

Sensory Cues

As the name implies, an external sensory cue is anything that prompts your desire to eat by targeting your senses. For example, you may smell your favorite meal or see a jar full of freshly baked cookies. You may even read a description of a meal in a magazine or watch a cooking show on television and start to feel hungry, even though you're not physically hungry. According to research, exposure to external sensory cues can significantly increase your desire to eat, even when your stomach is full and you're not truly hungry.

Social Cues

Although food is meant to be sustenance, it has become a way for people to entertain themselves and others. Going out to eat at a restaurant is now a favorite pastime, and you can rarely go to a party or other event without being offered all types of food. In many of these cases, it's likely that you'll eat even though you're not hungry; often you won't even realize it. In one study, published in the *American Journal of Health Behavior*, examining the effects of social cues on food consumption, undergraduate college students were instructed to eat alone and then instructed to eat with others. When these students ate with others, they consumed 60 percent more food than when they ate alone. Another study, published in the *Journal of Consumer Research*, showed that eating with a romantic partner can also affect the amount of food you take in. If one partner in the study ate more, the other was likely to eat more too.

Normative Cues

Normative cues are things like portion size or plate size, which affect the amount of food you eat. You may not even realize that you're being affected by these things, but research shows that when you use larger plates, you tend to serve yourself more and as a result you eat more.

Drink Up (Water, That Is)

During your fasting periods (and in general), water should be your best friend. You've probably heard that thirst is often mistaken for hunger, so staying hydrated can help diminish any false hunger signals. Right when you wake up, drink 8 ounces of water. You can prepare by having a glass of water on your nightstand when you go to sleep. Regularly sip water throughout the day and make sure to drink at least half of your body weight in ounces each day. If you exercise a lot or lose sweat in other ways, you may need to drink even more than that. You'll also need to add an extra glass of water for every cup of coffee or other diuretic you drink, so keep that in mind. The more hydrated you are, the less likely you'll experience false hunger signals.

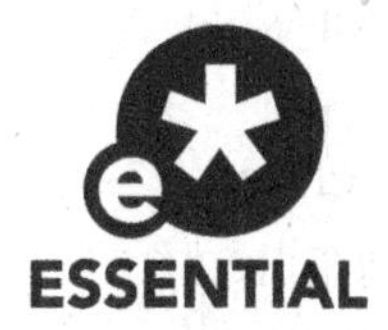

If drinking water isn't something that comes naturally to you, there are several apps you can download on your smartphone that can help. These apps allow you to set your water needs and will push a notification through to your phone periodically to remind you when it's time to drink up.

It might be helpful to buy a reusable water bottle that you really love. It may seem silly, but sometimes things just taste better when you're drinking them from certain containers. There are many companies out there that make stainless steel, insulated water bottles that keep your water cold for hours. You can refill these water bottles whenever necessary and bring them with you wherever you go so you always have clean water on hand. As an added bonus, using a reusable water bottle is better for the environment too.

Stay Busy

How many times have you thought you were hungry but it turned out you were just bored? One minute you're sitting around watching television and the next minute you're scouring through the pantry for something to snack on. Then, before you know it, an entire bag of chips is empty and you don't even know how it happened.

The best way to avoid this mindless snacking is to keep yourself—and your hands—occupied. Fill your schedule with fun and friends. Do creative projects or immerse yourself fully into work. If you feel boredom creeping in and you're tempted to eat just for the sake of eating, call a friend or a go for a walk around the neighborhood.

Look for (and Eliminate) Triggers

Look for things that trigger your psychological hunger—and then avoid those things. Up until now, you may have been on autopilot when it comes to eating. You haven't really been paying attention to what is going on around you or what is influencing the amount or the types of food you eat.

For example, do you have a significant other who eats twice as much as you do? Do you keep your favorite snacks in the pantry or refrigerator within sight every time you open the doors? Do you schedule social events around food? What kinds of restaurants are you choosing for these events, or what kinds of dishes are you and your friends making?

Figuring out the things that trigger you to eat more—or to choose unhealthy foods—will go a long way not only in maintaining intermittent fasting as a lifestyle but also in preserving your health. Surround yourself with people who support your lifestyle changes and stay away from—or limit time with—people who might sabotage your efforts.

Reduce Stress Levels

Stress is a major problem throughout the world. Approximately 77 percent of people in the United States report regularly feeling physical symptoms caused by stress, and 33 percent of those people say they are living with extreme stress. Stress can not only lead to weight gain but also heart disease, diabetes, headaches, depression, anxiety, and gastrointestinal problems.

One of the immediate ways stress contributes to weight gain is by tempting you to reach for comfort foods—like pizza or ice cream—which you may not crave when your stress levels are more under control. You've most likely heard of "emotional eating." Although some people tend to lose their appetite under high stress, many have an increased appetite for foods that are not conducive to a healthy lifestyle.

No matter which stress-eating category you fall into, you'll want to find ways to manage your stress. However, stress management is especially helpful in keeping hunger cues at bay if you fall into the latter category. Once your stress levels are under control, you'll be able to focus your attention on your eating plan and following the steps to help you reach your goals.

Sleep

The importance of sleep cannot be overstated—not just for staving off hunger but for your health in general. Sleep is nourishing and restorative, and when you don't get enough of it, it can completely throw you off in all areas. When you're stressed out, it's easy to skimp out on sleeping in favor of trying to knock a couple more things off of your to-do list, but don't do it!

Sleep time is when your brain and body repair and recharge, and it is vital to managing your stress levels and your hunger hormones. Sleep also contributes to increased mood and energy levels, ability to concentrate, and willpower—which is extremely important in the beginning stages of intermittent fasting.

There are two major hormones—ghrelin and leptin—involved in the hunger response. Ghrelin is the hunger hormone, and when it is released into your body, it tells your brain, "Hey, you're hungry; let's eat." Leptin is the satiation hormone, and it says, "Okay, you're satisfied now. You can stop eating." When you're sleep-deprived, the amount of ghrelin your body produces increases, while the amount of leptin it produces decreases. As a result, your body is constantly telling you that you're hungry and rarely, if ever, telling you that you're satisfied. In addition to this hormonal imbalance, your metabolism slows down when you're sleep-deprived, so you're not as efficiently burning off the food you're eating.

Always prioritize sleep. Make sure you're hitting the sheets by ten p.m. and getting seven to nine hours of uninterrupted sleep each night. Just like with your intermittent fasting plan, try to stick to the same sleep schedule (the same bedtime and wake-up time), even on the weekends. This helps regulate your circadian rhythm, just like fasting does. Make sure your room is dark and free from any unnecessary noises or lights, especially from electronic devices. Keep your phone in a different room or turn it off so any alerts won't disrupt your sleep. Put away all electronics at least one hour before bedtime. Watch your caffeine intake and switch to decaffeinated drinks after two p.m.

Be gentle with yourself and give it time; changing your eating and sleeping habits won't be easy right away, but if you give it your all, it will get much easier as time goes on.

Tips and Tools to Stay Focused

The most important thing you can do to ensure your success with intermittent fasting is to have a plan. The first step is to determine which type of fasting you're going to do. Once you've determined the type of fasting, make a schedule. Are you going to fast every day? What times will you fast and what times will you feed? After you've developed your timeline, another critical component is determining what you're going to eat when it's time to enter your fed state. Are you going to follow a specific dietary regimen (like the ketogenic diet or Paleo Diet) or are you going to stick to a basic clean-eating plan with no real "rules"?

Incorporate Meal Prep

Once you've got the basics down, prepping your meals can help keep you on track and prevent you from reaching for an unhealthy meal in times of hunger. Research shows that people who prepare their meals ahead of time experience greater success with their health and nutrition goals and also save time and money in the long run. As you get into the groove of intermittent fasting and your new way of eating, you can make adjustments to your meals and your prepping routine.

Meal-Prepping Tips

Getting organized is one of the most vital components of successful meal prep. It may seem daunting or like a waste of time to sit down and organize recipes and write everything out, but it will end up saving you time down the road.

The amount of meals you prepare in advance and the amount of time you spend cooking is completely up to you. Some people spend three or four hours on Sunday prepping meals for the entire week. Others spend a couple of hours on Sunday prepping meals for the next few days and then spend another couple of hours on Wednesday prepping meals for the rest of the week. Regardless of what style of meal prepping you choose, organization is key.

Figure Out Your Plan

First you'll need to design your meal plan. You can plan out a few days, a week, or even the entire month. Find simple recipes and write down everything you'll be eating and at what time. When you're first starting with intermittent fasting and meal planning, the excitement may tempt you to look for fancy, new recipes or a lot of variety, but when you're in the initial stages of a new lifestyle change, one of the most beneficial things you can do is stick to the basics and not overcomplicate things.

Stick to foods that you're already familiar with and recipes that won't take too long to prepare or that require you to learn new kitchen skills or buy new kitchen tools. There's plenty of time for you to try new things after you get used to the basics and your body and mind adjust to the changes. The point of meal prepping is to make you feel less overwhelmed, not add any unnecessary stress.

There are online meal planners and trackers as well as phone apps that you can use to keep track of your meals, but you don't need any fancy tools or software if technology isn't your thing. You can keep it simple by recording everything in a notebook.

Write Your Grocery List

Once you've gotten your recipes together and your meal plan written out, it's time to figure out what you need. Check your refrigerator and your pantry prior to writing your grocery list so you don't purchase things you already have. After you've compiled a list of things you have on hand, write out a grocery list of the remaining items you'll need to complete your recipes and your meals for the week (or for whatever length of time you've chosen).

You can save even more time by organizing your grocery list based on where items are found in the supermarket. You can list all meats together, all produce items together, and all refrigerated items together. If you need to go to different stores for any deals or any specialty items, organize your lists by store.

Make Your Meals

A great way to save time is to do your shopping on the same day you're going to make your meals. That way, you won't have to put as many grocery items away when you get home—you can jump right into making your meals. Once your meals are cooked, divide them into separate containers by portion sizes and label them appropriately. Now when you're ready to eat you'll have a meal ready to go, and if you're taking a meal with you on the go, it will be easy to transport.

Take Pictures and Measurements

If weight loss is one of your goals, don't rely solely on the scale. Your actual weight can fluctuate significantly from day to day, and you might not see big changes in the numbers even when your body is going through a massive transformation. You can use the scale as a tool, but take these day-to-day numbers with a grain of salt.

Instead, take "before" and "after" (or "progress") pictures. Down the line, you can compare them side by side to see how your body has changed over time. Pictures can be a really motivating tool because when you see yourself every day, you may not notice the small changes occurring, but when you compare pictures that were taken a month apart, the changes may be significantly more apparent. Don't let any current dissatisfaction with your body stop you from taking before pictures. You'll be happy you have them down the road.

In addition to pictures, it's helpful to take body measurements. You may start to build more lean muscle mass, especially if you're working out or strength training regularly. As your body starts to change, you may not notice too much of a shift on the scale, but your body composition can change dramatically. Measurements can help you track progress by documenting inches lost from different areas of your body. You'll want to take the following measurements:

- **Bust:** measure all the way around your bust, keeping the measuring tape in line with your nipples.
- **Chest:** measure directly underneath your breasts or pectoral muscles and all the way around your back.
- **Waist:** find the narrowest part of your waist, usually right below your ribcage, and measure all the way around.
- **Hips:** find the widest area of your hips and measure all the way around.
- **Thighs:** measure all the way around the fullest part of your upper leg while standing up straight.
- **Knees:** measure all the way around directly above the knee while standing up straight.
- **Upper arms:** measure all the way around the fullest part of your upper arms above your elbows.
- **Lower arms:** measure all the way around the fullest part of your lower arms below your elbows.

To properly measure, you'll need a nonstretchable measuring tape. Keep the tape level around your body and parallel to the floor. When you're taking your measurements, wrap the tape around your body as close to your skin as possible, but don't squeeze so tightly that the tape measure cuts into your skin or makes an indentation. It's helpful to have someone else take your measurements for you so you can stand straight; if you don't have someone available, take your measurements in front of a mirror to make sure that you're keeping the tape level and measuring in the correct spots.

Make a list of your measurements in a notebook or in your phone's notepad. Take your measurements every few weeks and record the numbers in the same place every time. As time passes, you can use the measurements to chart your progress.

Expect Ups and Downs

Like anything in life, you'll experience ups and downs with intermittent fasting, especially in the very beginning. Don't expect everything to go smoothly right off the bat and don't get caught up in perfection. You're going to slip up: you're going to eat outside of your feeding window sometimes, and that's okay. If you go into it knowing that you're going to put your best foot forward but also understanding that it can take a little while to get used to the transition, you'll be less likely to beat yourself up when things don't go totally according to plan.

CHAPTER 3

Health Benefits of Intermittent Fasting

One of the most common reasons people jump into intermittent fasting is weight loss, but that's barely scratching the surface. Intermittent fasting does so much more for your body than helping you shed pounds. It also helps stabilize your blood sugar levels, decease chronic or widespread inflammation, and improve your heart health. Studies have also shown that intermittent fasting may contribute to brain health, helping decrease your risk of developing major brain diseases like Alzheimer's.

Weight Loss

You've probably heard that if you eat less, you lose more weight—but what if weight loss has less to do with the amount of food you're eating and more to do with the amount of time during which you're eating it? When you hear how intermittent fasting works, you may think "Well, yeah, if you're eating during a smaller window of time, you'll be eating fewer calories, and that's why you lose weight." That's part of it: in some cases, you'll be eating fewer calories, especially because you'll be cutting out the late-night mindless snacking that can quickly contribute to weight gain. But that's not the whole story. Studies have shown that intermittent fasting can reduce weight and improve metabolism even without an overall calorie restriction.

One study published in *Translational Research* found that intermittent fasting can reduce body weight by 3–8 percent in a period of three to twenty-four weeks. The participants in this study also lost 4–7 percent of their waist circumference, which indicates that they lost belly fat—or visceral fat—which is the type of fat thought to be most dangerous to physical heath.

Visceral fat is the type of body fat that's stored deep inside the abdominal cavity. It lies in close proximity to several vital organs, including the liver, stomach, pancreas, and intestines. Having a lot of visceral fat is more dangerous than having extra subcutaneous fat (the fat that lies just underneath your skin) because visceral fat can affect your hormones and the way your body operates. It's linked to a greater risk of heart disease, cancer, stroke, diabetes, arthritis, obesity, and depression. There's no surefire way to tell if your fat is subcutaneous or visceral, but if you carry a lot of weight around your midsection, it's likely that you have a higher percentage of visceral fat.

Disproving Old Wisdom

The most common and persistent pieces of weight-loss advice are "eat less, move more" and "calories in versus calories out." The general principle underlying these weight-loss theories is that if you take in fewer calories than you burn off, you'll lose weight; but if you look at the statistics, these notions don't add up. For the past twenty years, people have been instructed to follow low-calorie, low-fat diets and to eat five to six small meals each day. Yet, during these twenty years, obesity rates have increased substantially. Of course, there's the argument that people simply just aren't putting in the work required to lose weight, but in many cases this isn't true. There are scores of people who exercise regularly and eat "healthily" yet still have nothing to show for it. This is because weight loss isn't that simple—and conventional wisdom has been proven wrong.

In the early 1970s, 14 percent of the United States population was classified as obese. Today, more than one in three, or 39.8 percent, of American adults are obese. Approximately one in five, or 18.5 percent, of children and adolescents in the United States between the ages of two and nineteen are considered obese. Some of the leading causes of preventable death, such as heart disease, stroke, certain types of cancer, and type 2 diabetes, are linked to obesity.

One study, called the Women's Health Initiative, followed approximately fifty thousand women for a period of almost eight years. During that time, one-half of the women followed a low-fat, low-calorie diet and increased their exercise output by 14 percent. This group was classified as the intervention group. The second half of the women followed their usual diet and exercise routine. The average difference in weight loss in the intervention group after almost eight years? Less than 2 pounds.

Studies also show that people who follow dietary plans, like intermittent fasting, that allow a greater variability in food choices are more likely to stick to the diet and maintain weight loss than those who follow a rigid, calorie-controlled diet. Rigid diets are also associated with symptoms of disordered eating and a higher BMI (or Body Mass Index, which is measure of your body fat using weight and height) in nonobese women, while flexible dieting strategies, like intermittent fasting, are not.

Hearing this may be discouraging, especially if you've subscribed to the theory that the way to lose weight is to restrict calories and exercise more—but this is actually good news. You don't have to spend your days counting calories, eating too little, and avoiding healthy fats. There's a better way: intermittent fasting.

How Intermittent Fasting Helps You Lose Weight

While intermittent fasting does naturally help you cut calories (even without calorie counting), it contributes to weight loss in other ways by helping to balance several growth hormones that have an effect on the way you lose and retain weight. Studies show that short-term fasting can also boost your metabolism by as much 14 percent. On the other hand, fasts that last more than forty-eight hours can negatively affect metabolism.

The Effect on Human Growth Hormone

Human growth hormone, or HGH, is a naturally occurring hormone that's produced by your pituitary gland—a small endocrine gland in your brain that also controls your adrenals and thyroid. When your body releases HGH, it stays in the bloodstream, where the liver converts it into other active growth factors, such as insulin-like growth factor, or IGF-1. These growth factors promote growth in every cell of your body. When you fast, the levels of human growth hormone in your body naturally increase. In fact, some research shows that the levels can increase as much as five times when compared to times you don't fast.

Supplementing an outside source of human growth hormone is not recommended. Your body doesn't recognize this human growth hormone in the same way that it recognizes the substance your brain naturally produces. Side effects of using supplemental human growth hormone include nerve and muscle pain, swelling, carpal tunnel syndrome, numbness and tingling of the skin, and high cholesterol levels. Using supplemental human growth hormone can also increase the risk of developing diabetes and contribute to the growth of cancerous tumors.

One of the most notable benefits of human growth hormone is its ability to stimulate the synthesis of collagen in both the skeletal muscles and tendons. When the muscles and tendons contain more collagen, it results in increased muscle strength, which can improve your physical capabilities and exercise performance. When you have more muscle mass, it also increases your basal metabolic rate. This makes your body more efficient at using up calories, even when you're not active. Human growth hormone also increases lipolysis—a physiological process during which fat and triglycerides are broken apart and turned into free fatty acids, which are then removed from the body. An increase in lipolysis translates to easier and faster weight loss.

One study published in *The Journal of Clinical Endocrinology & Metabolism* showed that human growth hormone can help reduce abdominal and visceral fat, specifically. This same study also reported improvements in both blood pressure and insulin sensitivity in participants.

The Impact on Norepinephrine

Norepinephrine, also referred to as noradrenaline, is a neurotransmitter that is released by the sympathetic nervous system in times of stress. Thus, it's also classified as a stress hormone. When levels of norepinephrine in the body go up, it triggers an increase in heart rate, a release of glucose into the blood, and an increase in blood flow to the muscles. Norepinephrine also speeds up reaction time and increases alertness and awareness.

Since fasting is a stressor, it signals your body to release norepinephrine, which also acts on fat cells, breaking them down into free fatty acids. In the absence of glucose (due to fasting) your body then turns to these free fatty acids for energy, burning them up and reducing your body fat as a result.

Your autonomic nervous system is categorized into two parts: sympathetic and parasympathetic. The sympathetic nervous system kicks on in times of stress or distress. It's characterized by increased sweating, reduced blood flow, dilated pupils, and dry mouth. The parasympathetic nervous system, also known as "rest and digest," is activated when you're relaxed. Activation of the parasympathetic nervous system is characterized by a decrease in heart rate, relaxed muscles, dilated blood vessels, and a decrease in pupil size.

Insulin and Glucose Balance

Your body obtains energy from three main sources, called the macronutrients: carbohydrates, fat, and protein—in that order. The ingestion of these macronutrients causes a rise in both glucose and insulin, but the degree at which these levels rise differs based on which one you're eating and how much of it you are eating.

Carbohydrates, especially refined carbohydrates and simple sugars, cause the most substantial increases in both glucose and insulin, whereas fat and protein cause more moderate increases. This is significant because the rises in blood sugar and insulin affect the way you use the sugar and the hormone. The way your body responds to insulin says a lot about your ability to lose weight and your health in general.

One of insulin's main jobs is to move glucose from your bloodstream into your cells, where it's used as energy, or to move it to the liver, where it's converted to glycogen and stored for later use. If you are resistant to insulin, your body doesn't respond to normal amounts of insulin properly, and instead of moving to your cells, glucose and insulin remain in the bloodstream. When glucose and insulin stay floating in your blood, the pancreas releases even more insulin in an effort to lower your glucose (blood sugar) levels. High insulin levels are connected to a reduced ability to burn fat—in other words, difficulty losing weight. But what causes insulin resistance and how can you reverse it? Fasting.

Statistics show that approximately sixty to seventy million adults are affected by insulin resistance. If not corrected, insulin resistance can destroy the beta cells (the cells responsible for producing and releasing insulin) in the pancreas and contribute to the develop of prediabetes and diabetes. The American Diabetes Association (ADA) estimates that 70 percent of those with insulin resistance will go on to develop type 2 diabetes if significant lifestyle changes aren't made.

The way to help correct insulin resistance is to lower the amount of insulin that your body is producing—and you can do this by eating less. When you eat, the levels of glucose and insulin in your body rise. As a result, your body starts burning off glucose for energy instead of fat. When you don't eat, glucose and insulin levels stay lower, and your body turns to stored fat for energy—ultimately resulting in weight loss.

What about Low-Carb Diets?

Low-carb diets are developed around the physiology of insulin and its effect on the way your body burns fat. Because of this, low-carb diets can help reverse insulin resistance, but some people may need an extra push. Again, all macronutrients (carbohydrates, fat, and protein) raise your glucose and insulin levels to some degree, so abstaining from food completely for periods of time can have a more powerful effect on insulin resistance than restricting carbohydrates alone.

Improved Blood Sugar Regulation

Although weight loss is a welcome side effect of getting your blood sugar levels under control, it's not the only benefit. Insulin resistance and chronically high blood sugar put you at risk of developing type 2 diabetes and the complications that come with it. Using fasting as a tool to help balance your blood sugar levels will improve your health and prevent you from entering—or remove you from—the diabetes "danger zone."

The Prevalence of Diabetes

According to the 2017 *National Diabetes Statistics Report* released by the Centers for Disease Control and Prevention, approximately 30.3 million Americans are currently living with diabetes, and 7.2 million of them are undiagnosed cases. Another 84.1 million adults (almost 34 percent of the adult US population) are living with prediabetes.

When you fast and teach your body to burn fat for energy instead of glucose, it not only lowers insulin and blood sugar levels but also improves insulin sensitivity. Balanced blood sugar levels are also associated with:

- Improved fasting blood glucose (blood sugar levels after going twelve hours without eating)

- Improved postprandial blood glucose (blood sugar levels after eating a meal)
- Reduced glucose variability (drastic increases and dips in blood sugar levels)

Reduced glucose variability is especially notable when it comes to concerns with hunger. When you get hungry after a short period of time without food, it's often because your blood sugar dips dramatically after an increase. This is because your pancreas releases a rush of insulin in response to the presence of glucose in your blood. When the insulin rushes into your blood and carries the glucose into your cells, it results in a decrease in blood sugar. This decrease is the cause of hunger and any uncomfortable symptoms that come with it. The greater the initial spike in blood sugar, the greater the resulting dip will be.

When you fast, there are no rapid increases in blood sugar, which means there are no dramatic decreases either. As a result, you'll experience less hunger and you'll avoid the other symptoms of low blood sugar, which include:

- Dizziness or light-headedness
- Irritability
- Anxiety
- Increased sweating
- Fatigue
- Shakiness
- Confusion
- Dry mouth
- Headache
- Blurred vision

Of course, it may take some time for your body to adjust to your new lifestyle and for your blood sugar levels to regulate. Because of this, you may experience some symptoms of low blood sugar when you first start your fasting regimen.

Decreased Inflammation

Inflammation is another largely misunderstood physiological response in the body. You often hear the word *inflammation* used in a negative way, but it's actually an important immune reaction that is one of the body's most vital protective mechanisms. Without inflammation, no infections, cuts, or other damage to the skin would be able to heal. That being said, inflammation can be divided into two categories: acute and chronic. Acute inflammation is the beneficial type, while chronic inflammation can cause long-term health problems.

Acute Inflammation versus Chronic Inflammation

When you get a cut or an infection like the flu, inflammation can save your life. In response to the threat, the small branches of your arteries enlarge, which results in increased blood flow to the affected area. Then your immune system sends out white blood cells, called neutrophils, that contain enzymes to break down the infection or wound. These neutrophils surround the affected area and create redness and swelling, which protects the area and the rest of the body until the immediate threat goes away. This process is called acute inflammation. Symptoms of acute inflammation include:

- Pain at the injury site
- Redness
- Swelling
- Heat
- Immobility

These five symptoms are most noticeable when inflammation occurs on the skin, but the same process happens internally when your body is fighting an infection that you can't see, such as a cold. Acute inflammation typically lasts for a few days.

The opposite of acute inflammation is chronic inflammation, which is where the trouble with inflammation lies. Unlike acute inflammation, which is short-lasting, chronic inflammation is ongoing. Your body experiences chronic inflammation in response to a prolonged threat. The trouble is that the threat is not often obvious, and that's why chronic inflammation is often dubbed the "silent killer." You may experience chronic inflammation in response to a pathogen that the body cannot break down, such as a stubborn virus that remains in your system, an overactive immune response from an undiagnosed food sensitivity, or a toxin from your environment. Chronic inflammation can also arise from prolonged, unmanaged stress or nutrient deficiencies. Whatever the cause, chronic inflammation can be dangerous to your health. Unlike acute inflammation, which typically goes away after a few days, chronic inflammation can last from several months to a number of years. If chronic inflammation is left untreated, it can cause thickening and scarring of connective tissue and even result in tissue death. Some conditions associated with chronic inflammation include:

- Heart disease
- Stroke
- Cancer
- Chronic respiratory diseases, like asthma
- Obesity
- Diabetes
- Ulcerative colitis and Crohn's disease
- Neurological diseases
- Autoimmune diseases

Statistics from The National Institutes of Health estimate that 23.5–50 million Americans suffer from some type of autoimmune disease, which is the term for any condition in which the immune system mistakenly attacks itself and your own body. Research is unclear on what exactly causes autoimmune disease to develop, but chronic inflammation is thought to be a major risk factor.

Many people with chronic inflammation don't even realize they have it for a while, because it doesn't always cause symptoms. When symptoms do develop, they may include:

- Fatigue
- Persistent low-grade fever

- Rashes, eczema, or psoriasis
- Joint or muscle pain
- Abdominal pain
- Excess weight around the midsection
- Digestive issues (gas, bloating, diarrhea, constipation)
- Allergies
- Puffy face and/or puffy bags under the eyes
- Depression or anxiety
- Brain fog
- Gum disease

How Fasting Reduces Chronic Inflammation

Fasting can help reduce chronic inflammation through several different mechanisms. Leukotrienes are biologically active molecules that are formed by leukocytes (a type of white blood cells). They are pro-inflammatory and play a major role in asthma attacks, allergic diseases, and anaphylaxis, which is a severe, potentially fatal allergic reaction. Leukotrienes are also involved in a wide variety of other diseases. While small amounts of leukotrienes are helpful for acute inflammation, higher levels contribute to chronic inflammation.

One study published in *Arthritis & Rheumatology* on individuals with rheumatoid arthritis (a degenerative disease of the joints that's connected to chronic inflammation) found that fasting not only reduced the amount of leukotrienes in the body but it also changed the phospholipid (a type of fat that's a major component of your cell membranes) fatty acid composition of the cell membranes. This is significant because the phospholipid composition plays a role in generating the precursors to specific leukotrienes.

Another way that fasting helps reduce chronic inflammation is by acting on inflammatory cytokines. Cytokines are small proteins that have a specific effect on the communication between cells. Cytokines can be either anti-inflammatory or pro-inflammatory. The pro-inflammatory cytokines have been shown to not only turn on sensory neurons that cause pain but also to play a part in keeping that pain response turned on. In other words, if pro-inflammatory cytokines are constantly released into your body, you'll experience chronic pain. Certain pro-inflammatory cytokines are also linked to allodynia—the pain associated with conditions like fibromyalgia and migraines. Allodynia is described as an unusual pain response to stimuli that doesn't typically cause pain, such as someone lightly touching your skin or brushing your hair. Studies show that combining fasting with calorie restriction can reduce the production and release of pro-inflammatory cytokines, thus reducing chronic inflammation and persistent pain.

Through separate studies, researchers at Yale University found that when you fast, your body produces a compound that can block the part of the immune system that's involved in various inflammatory disorders. These blocked receptors and sensors, known as inflammasomes, are connected to a number of different inflammatory disorders. Research shows that inflammasomes are at least partly responsible for the development and progression of metabolic diseases, like diabetes and nonalcoholic fatty liver disease, and neurodegenerative diseases, like Parkinson's disease, dementia, and Huntington's disease.

When you fast, your body produces a compound called beta-hydroxybutyrate, or BHB. BHB acts directly on a certain inflammasome called NLRP3, shutting off the inflammatory response and reducing the negative effects of chronic inflammation on the body.

BHB is technically classified as a ketone. It makes up approximately 78 percent of the body's ketones, while acetoacetate (AcAc) and acetone make up the remaining 22 percent. BHB is extremely stable and plentiful, so it's the ketone used most frequently for energy. In addition to fasting, you can increase the amount of BHB in your body by following a ketogenic (or high-fat, low-carbohydrate diet), restricting calories without causing malnutrition, and engaging in high-intensity exercise.

Fasting also promotes autophagy—the process during which the body destroys old and/or damaged cells and stimulates their removal. When old and damaged cells remain in the body, it can stimulate chronic inflammation because your body attacks these cells. When autophagy is stimulated, the removal of these cells helps to turn off that unnecessary inflammation.

Eating to Ease Inflammation

In addition to fasting, there are certain foods that have been shown to help reduce chronic inflammation, so if you suspect that you're dealing with chronic inflammation, you may want to include them in your diet. These foods include:

- Olive oil
- Nuts
- Leafy greens
- Fatty fish, like salmon and mackerel
- Tomatoes
- Fruit, especially blueberries

On the other hand, certain foods have been shown to aggravate inflammation, so it may be best to avoid these:

- Fried foods
- Refined carbohydrates (white bread, white rice, desserts)
- Sugar (including soda and sweetened drinks)
- Margarine
- Factory-farmed red meat

A Healthier Heart

In the United States, heart disease is the leading cause of death for both men and women. Every year, approximately 610,000 deaths (which averages out to about one in four American deaths) are attributed to heart disease. The American Heart Association asserts that the biggest contributor to these statistics is the lack of commitment to a heart-healthy lifestyle. In other words, many cases of heart disease develop due to risk factors that you can control. One of these major risk factors is your diet.

Although medical experts agree that a heart-healthy lifestyle can help lower your risk of heart disease, there is some disagreement about what that lifestyle actually entails. There is a pervasive myth that one of the best things you can do for your heart is follow a low-fat, low-cholesterol diet, even though research has disproven this time and time again. To fully understand how intermittent fasting contributes to a healthier heart, you need a little background on cholesterol.

The Cholesterol Myth

Cholesterol has developed a really bad reputation, but the lipoprotein—as cholesterol is physiologically classified—is largely misunderstood. Cholesterol performs three major functions in your body, and without it, you wouldn't be able to survive. It's a component of the bile acids that help you digest fats; it's a major piece of the outer layer of every one of your cells; and it's also an important part of vitamin D and certain hormones like estrogen and testosterone.

There are two major types of cholesterol: LDL and HDL. LDL cholesterol is categorized as "bad" cholesterol, while HDL is classified as "good" cholesterol. Many cholesterol tests also measure triglycerides. While not technically cholesterol, triglycerides are another type of fat in your blood that is used to store extra energy—or calories—from the food you eat. High levels of triglycerides are associated with both heart disease and insulin resistance.

When you get a standard cholesterol test—or "lipid profile"—your doctor looks at all the numbers: your total cholesterol, LDL cholesterol, and HDL cholesterol. If the values for total cholesterol and/or LDL cholesterol are elevated, it's considered a risk factor for developing heart disease.

Despite a common misconception, the cholesterol you eat has a minimal impact on the amount of cholesterol in your blood. This is because your body doesn't absorb dietary cholesterol well. Most of the cholesterol you get from your diet travels right through your digestive system and never even makes it into your blood. Another reason your body doesn't absorb cholesterol well is because it is good at controlling cholesterol levels. When you eat a lot of cholesterol, the natural production of cholesterol in your liver slows down to balance it out. Only about 20 percent of the cholesterol in your blood comes from the food you eat. The remaining 80 percent is produced directly by your liver. Your body is designed to have a certain amount of cholesterol, so if you're limiting the cholesterol in your diet, your liver will ramp up its production to compensate. This means that if you eat one egg per day, which contains 200–300 milligrams of cholesterol, your liver will produce an additional 800 milligrams from the fats, sugars, and proteins already in your body.

Additionally, while high LDL cholesterol is considered a risk factor for heart disease, it's not the numbers that matter as much as the size of the LDL particles. Some LDL particles are small, hard, and dense. These particles are the ones that stick to your arterial walls and cause the buildup of plaque that's associated with heart disease, heart attacks, and stroke. Other LDL particles are large and fluffy. These LDL particles bounce around your arteries, never sticking to the walls—and thus, never causing a problem. If your LDL levels are high but most of the LDL particles are the large, fluffy kind, your risk of heart disease diminishes.

Fasting's Effect on Cholesterol Levels

Intermittent fasting can reduce total cholesterol levels by as much as 20 percent; but what's even more impressive than that is the effect intermittent fasting has on individual lipids. Studies show that an eight-week alternate day fast can reduce LDL cholesterol levels by approximately 25 percent. Fasting also reduces the number of the small, dense LDL particles. When the body is not making new free fatty acids (like when you are on a fasting plan), it results in a decrease of VLDL, or very low-density lipoproteins, which in turn, reduces LDL.

That's not all: fasting can also decrease triglycerides by as much as 32 percent; and while it lowers both problematic cholesterol markers, fasting has no negative effect on HDL, or "good" cholesterol.

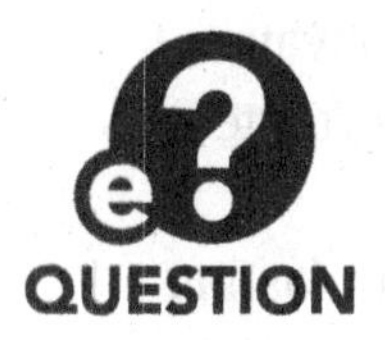

What are very low-density lipoproteins?
Lipoproteins, which carry cholesterol, triglycerides, and other fats through the body, are compounds made up of cholesterol, triglycerides, and proteins. They are separated into different categories based on the ratio of each of these three components that they contain. Very low-density lipoproteins contain the highest amounts of triglycerides. These lipoproteins are characterized as "bad cholesterol" because they can accumulate on the walls of your arteries and contribute to the development of heart disease.

A Healthier Brain

Fatigue, brain fog, and an inability to concentrate are some of the most common symptoms plaguing people today; but although these symptoms are common, they're not normal in a properly functioning body. High blood sugar and insulin levels, insulin resistance, and excess weight all contribute to decreased brain function. Because intermittent fasting helps balance blood sugar and insulin levels—and can help you shed excess pounds—it also leads to marked improvement in these symptoms. But intermittent fasting doesn't just positively affect your brain by balancing your blood sugar levels; it can have more direct effects on your brain health through several other mechanisms.

According to Dr. Mark Mattson, a professor of neuroscience at Johns Hopkins University, intermittent fasting has been shown to increase the rate of neurogenesis (the development of new brain cells and nerve tissues in the brain). Increased rates of neurogenesis are linked with boosts in mood, memory, focus, and overall brain function.

Intermittent fasting also increases the production of a protein called brain-derived neurotrophic factor, or BDNF, which plays a number of roles in your brain and general health. When your brain is challenged—by anything from intense exercise or mental stimulation to calorie restriction—the body increases its production of BDNF. A higher level of BDNF not only strengthens the connection between existing neurons but also increases the brain's production of new neurons. Furthermore, high levels of BDNF are associated with lower levels of depression and a boost in mood and motivation. One study published in the *Journal of Neurochemistry* found that intermittent fasting can increase BDNF levels by as much as 400 percent.

The increase in human growth hormone caused by intermittent fasting has also been shown to improve cognition, protect the brain from damage, and increase the production of new brain cells.

CHAPTER 4

Types of Intermittent Fasting

There are several types of intermittent fasting, and while some methods are more popular than others, the best method for you depends on your schedule and how your body reacts. All types of fasting stimulate autophagy (a process during which your body cleans out old or destroyed compounds that can cause disease or illness), which is the goal. In order to be successful with intermittent fasting, you'll have to be able to stick to it, so the best thing to do is pick the type of intermittent fasting that best fits your current routine. When you're just starting out, you may want to experiment with the different methods to see which type works best for you, then adjust based on how you feel.

Fasting and Autophagy

Autophagy is a normal physiological process that is involved in cleaning out old or destroyed compounds in the body. Although it sounds a little unnerving, the literal translation of autophagy is "self-eating." It's derived from the Greek words *autos*, which translates to "self," and *phagein*, which means "to eat." The term *autophagy* was coined by Christian de Duve, a Nobel Prize–winning scientist, after a group of researchers noticed an increase in lysosomes (the parts of the cells responsible for breaking down and destroying other compounds) in liver cells after injections of glucagon, the hormone that works in opposition to insulin.

Autophagy plays a key role in maintaining homeostasis—a stable and healthy internal environment—in the body. Your body constantly has proteins and organelles (small, specialized structures in each of your body's cells) that become dysfunctional or die. If allowed to accumulate in the body, these dead tissues can cause cell death, contribute to poor tissue and/or organ function, and even become cancerous. During autophagy, the body marks damaged parts of cells and unused proteins in the body. These damaged parts are sent to the lysosomes, where they're cleared out of the body. This process prevents them from causing harm.

Dr. Colin Champ, a board-certified radiation oncologist and assistant professor at the University of Pittsburgh Medical Center, describes this process as an innate recycling program. He claims that the process of autophagy makes your body more efficient by removing any faulty parts, stopping any metabolic dysfunction (like obesity and diabetes), and stopping cancerous (and potentially cancerous) growths.

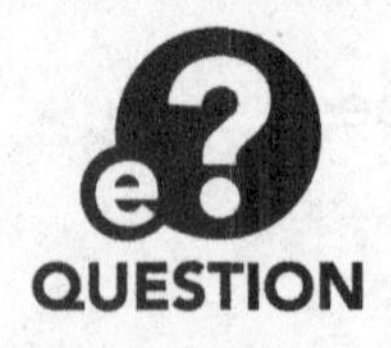

What happens without autophagy?

When autophagy is not "turned on," dead proteins remain in the body and start to accumulate. These dead proteins are associated with the development of chronic diseases, most notably Alzheimer's disease and cancer. Alzheimer's disease is characterized by the buildup by one or two of these proteins—amyloid beta or tau protein—which accumulate in the brain and contribute to the plaques associated with the conditions.

There's also evidence that autophagy may play a role in decreasing chronic inflammation and boosting natural immunity. Research shows that subjects who are not capable of inducing autophagy tend to carry more weight, sleep more often, and have higher cholesterol levels and decreased brain function.

Fasting is one of the most effective ways to stimulate autophagy in both the body and the brain, because depriving the body of certain nutrients for a set period of time turns the process on. When insulin goes up (after eating), glucagon (the hormone that acts opposite to insulin) goes down. Conversely, when insulin goes down (after a period without food), glucagon goes up. When you fast, glucagon increases, stimulating autophagy.

After a period of fasting, the number of autophagosomes—the organelles responsible for clearing the cellular waste—increases significantly in the body. Some studies found that the amount of autophagosomes can go up by as much as 300 percent after fasting.

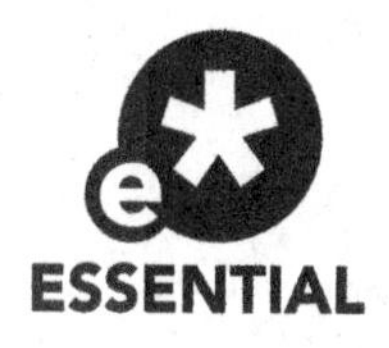

Many people go on juice cleanses or juice fasts in an effort to cleanse the body, but depending on what's in the juice, this could actually work against you. Juices that contain high-sugar fruit or high-carbohydrate vegetables will raise insulin enough so that glucagon goes down, which will prevent autophagy and the cellular cleansing that comes with it. Fresh, low-sugar juices can be an excellent source of micronutrients, however.

While the science is clear that fasting increases autophagy, the one thing that researchers don't agree on is exactly how to fast to maximize the process. Each of the fasting methods has been shown to stimulate autophagy, and no single method has been proven to be better than another. Each method has its own pros and cons, so ultimately it's up to you to decide which protocol works best for you.

The 16/8 Method

The 16/8 method of fasting, also known as the Leangains protocol, is the most popular type of intermittent fasting. It was originally developed by

Martin Berkhan, a nutritional expert and personal trainer who was looking for a way to help his clients build muscle without accumulating fat. When following the 16/8 method, you schedule a sixteen-hour fasting window and an eight-hour feeding window each day. This means that you'll go for sixteen hours without eating anything, fitting all of your meals within a consecutive eight-hour time frame. For example, you may choose a fasting window between seven p.m. and eleven a.m., which means the feeding window would fall between eleven a.m. and seven p.m.

There are no hard rules about the times you must eat, but once you decide on a schedule, you'll want to stick to it every day. Berkhan says that if you don't have a consistent feeding window, it can throw your hormones out of whack and make it even harder to stick to the program because you'll experience more hunger and may not notice any of the positive health benefits. There are also no restrictions on the amount of meals you eat: you can fit breakfast, lunch, dinner, and even some snacks into the eight-hour eating window. Of course, if weight loss is one of your goals, you'll want to be more mindful of your calorie intake.

Research shows that women may do better with a fourteen- or fifteen-hour fasting window and a nine- or ten-hour eating window. If you're a woman and you want to follow the 16/8 method, start with a fourteen-hour fast and see how you feel. Easing in to it will give your hormones time to adjust and will make any negative side effects, like changes in or loss of energy, less likely.

During your fasting window, you are allowed to drink water, coffee, and other noncaloric beverages, such as tea or seltzer; however, pay attention to your caffeine intake and be careful not to overdo it. While sipping beverages during your fasting window can help stave off hunger, too much caffeine can leave you anxious, jittery, and dehydrated, especially when your stomach is empty. Caffeine also puts stress on your adrenals, so while your body is adjusting to the added stress of fasting, it's best to keep your coffee intake minimal.

One of the major benefits of this method of intermittent fasting is that it's fairly easy to incorporate into your schedule. Since you'll be sleeping for around eight hours of your fast, you only have to skip food for a small portion of your waking hours. Most people can successfully pull off the 16/8 method by not eating after dinner and then skipping breakfast or eating it late in the morning.

The science behind the 16/8 method is based on your biological clock and circadian rhythms. According to Satchidananda Panda, a professor at the Salk Institute for Biological Studies and an expert in the field of biology and circadian rhythms, the body doesn't just have one biological clock but rather several that make up the complete circadian rhythm. According to Panda, there's one biological clock in your liver, one in your kidneys, and one in your gut, and each of these clocks get turned on and turned off at different times.

When you eat, your digestive system immediately kicks into gear. As food moves through your digestive tract, each organ involved in the digestive process turns on, processes the food, and then turns off. When all of the digestive organs are turned off, the digestive system has time to rest. It's during this time that the digestive system does its own "cleanup"—similar to the concept of a self-cleaning oven. All the leftover food particles get washed out, and your body is ready to start fresh.

However, if you're constantly putting food into your body, your digestive system never shuts down, so it never has adequate time to perform its self-cleaning, which negatively affects both your digestion and your overall health. During his research, Panda found that giving your body an eight-to-twelve-hour window without food is ideal for your health. He proposes that incorporating a fasting window every day can help you lose weight (or maintain a heathy weight) and help stave off diabetes, high cholesterol, and obesity.

The Importance of Your Circadian Rhythm

To fully understand Panda's research, it's helpful to know what your circadian rhythm is and how it affects your body. Also referred to as a body clock or a biological clock, your circadian rhythm is a twenty-four-hour cycle that regulates many of your body's physiological processes, like sleep and digestion. Your body receives cues from your circadian rhythm about when to go to sleep, when to wake up, and when to eat.

Your circadian rhythm is controlled internally by an area of your brain called the hypothalamus, but it's largely affected by external, environmental cues like temperature and light. For example, when it's dark outside, your eyes send a signal to your hypothalamus that it's time to sleep; your hypothalamus sends a message to the pineal gland (in another area of the brain) to release melatonin (a hormone that helps you sleep), and you get tired. When it's light out, the opposite happens. Your eyes send a signal to your hypothalamus, which sends a signal to your pineal gland to decrease the production of melatonin. This dip in melatonin helps wake you up and prepare you for the day.

Many people take melatonin supplements to help with sleep because it is a natural supplement. While it's true that melatonin is natural, it's also a hormone, and care should be taken when using melatonin supplements. If you take them too often and for too long, it can throw off your hormonal balance and your body's natural circadian rhythm. If you're having trouble sleeping, try diffusing lavender essential oil as an alternative to melatonin supplements.

Your circadian rhythm is also affected by the timing of your meals. In the Paleolithic era, food was available mostly during daylight hours. This is because food needed to be hunted and gathered, and it was easier to do this during the day. Biologically, the human body prefers this cycle and has yet to properly adjust to the changes brought about by the Industrial Revolution and modern conveniences like grocery stores and artificial lighting.

In one study published in *Obesity*, participants were given either a large breakfast in the morning or a large dinner at night after the sun went down. The overall calorie intake of both groups was the same. At the end of the study, researchers found that the group given a large dinner later in the day had a much more significant rise in insulin than the group given a large breakfast in the morning. Researchers concluded that this effect is seen because insulin sensitivity and glucose tolerance decreases throughout the day. In other words, your body doesn't tolerate increases in blood sugar at night as well as it does earlier in the morning.

Although there isn't a specific diet you must follow while doing the 16/8 method, Berkhan recommends that whole, unprocessed foods make up the majority of your calorie intake. In addition to eating as cleanly as possible, you should incorporate protein as a moderate portion of your calorie intake.

On the days you exercise, most of the calories you don't take in from protein should be from carbohydrates. On rest days, fat intake should be higher than carbohydrate intake.

The Warrior Diet

The Warrior Diet, which was developed by Ori Hofmekler, a member of the Israeli Special Forces, is credited with being the catalyst to other intermittent fasting methods. Hofmekler introduced the Warrior Diet in 2001, after spending time in the army and studying the behavior and dietary patterns of the warrior societies of Rome and Sparta. He designed the Warrior Diet based on the belief that it was the natural way to eat before the Industrial Revolution and that following it could promote both weight loss and increased energy.

The Warrior Diet takes the 16/8 method one step further by extending the fasting period to closer to twenty hours. While following the Warrior Diet, you eat only one large meal at night. During the day, you can have light snacks—like berries, yogurt, and whey protein—as well as water, vegetable juices, coffee, and tea. Hofmekler describes the fasting part of the Warrior Diet as the "undereating" phase, and the four-hour feeding window as the "overeating" phase.

According to Hofmekler, the "undereating" phase takes place during the day because the stress of less food triggers the sympathetic nervous system's fight-or-flight response. As a result, you experience a boost in energy, a rise in adrenaline (which promotes alertness), and an increase in fat burning. The "overeating" phase takes place at night because the goal during this phase is to do the opposite of the "undereating" phase by triggering the parasympathetic nervous system's rest-and-digest response. When the body is in rest-and-digest mode, it promotes calmness and relaxation, improves digestion, and helps the body recuperate from the stresses of the day. When the body is relaxed, it's also able to use the nutrients you take in more efficiently.

Unlike other fasting methods, which don't specify exactly what types of food to eat during your feeding period, the Warrior Diet restricts certain combinations of food. For example, while following the Warrior Diet, you can combine protein and vegetables but must avoid combining nuts and fruits, grains and fruits, protein and grains, and alcohol and starch. The theory behind this is that your body is able to digest certain combinations of foods better than others. Combining protein and vegetables is easy on digestion, while combining protein with grains makes digestion more difficult.

During your four-hour eating window, you'll start by eating nonstarchy vegetables, protein, and fat. Once that settles, you can add in some carbohydrates if you're still hungry. The theory behind this is that eating in this pattern can optimize hormone production and the way your body burns fat during the day.

The Warrior Diet doesn't just focus on intermittent fasting, though: the true Warrior Diet also requires regular exercise during your fasted state. According to research, you can burn up to 20 percent more fat when you exercise in a fasted state. The theory is that high insulin levels can suppress the way your body metabolizes fat. When you fast, your insulin levels drop. If you activate your metabolism by exercising when insulin levels are low, you'll be able to burn more fat.

Eat Stop Eat

The Eat Stop Eat fasting protocol was developed by Brad Pilon, who designed the program after his graduate research at the University of Guelph in Canada. His goal was to develop a plan that helped people lose fat and gain muscle, without stress, obsessing over what to eat, or becoming overly fixated on healthy eating and exercise.

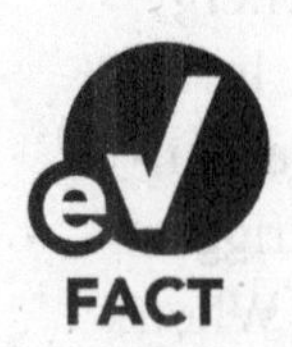

There are many drinks that are calorie-free but sweetened with artificial sweeteners. Although these are technically permitted during your fasting windows, they're not the best choices. Artificial sweeteners can disrupt your hunger hormones and make your cravings for sugary foods and drinks more intense. Some artificial sweeteners have also been connected with irritable bowel syndrome, certain cancers, obesity, diarrhea, gas and bloating, and migraines.

Instead of fasting every day, the Eat Stop Eat method involves incorporating a twenty-four-hour fast for either one or two days per week, and then eating normally on the other five or six days. With the Eat Stop Eat method, you choose the days and times of your fasts, but you must make sure that you're not eating for a full twenty-four hours. For example, your schedule may be to eat normally on Tuesday through Sunday, but to fast from Sunday night at eight p.m. to Monday night at eight p.m. Like with the 16/8 method, you cannot eat any food during your fasting windows, but you're allowed to drink calorie-free beverages. When your fast is over, you go back to eating normally.

Pilon believes that you're taught from a young age that you have to eat at certain times, and this idea can put a strain on you and on how you feel about eating in general. He defines intermittent fasting as the ability to practice patience when it comes to eating—or a conscious yet polite restraint. His philosophy is that "we do not have to eat all the time, therefore we are free to choose when we eat."

Because most of the focus on the Eat Stop Eat method is on meal timing, Pilon doesn't define any foods as forbidden or off-limits. You don't have to count calories or restrict your diet, and not doing either makes it easier to follow on feeding days, but if you want optimal results or your goal is to lose weight, you'll have to make smart choices when it comes to what you're eating.

The Eat Stop Eat method may be a little more difficult than the 16/8 method at first because you'll go full days without eating. If you're new to intermittent fasting, you may want to start with a type of intermittent fasting that has shorter fasting windows before moving to one that incorporates twenty-four-hour fasts.

The 5:2 Method

The 5:2 method, also called the Fast Diet, was made popular by Michael Mosley, a British physician and journalist. Like the Eat Stop Eat method, the 5:2 method involves fasting only on certain days of the week. With this method of fasting, you don't ever completely abstain from eating: you eat normally on five days of the week and then restrict calories to 500–600 per day on the other two days of the week.

For example, while following the 5:2 method, you may eat normally on Monday, Wednesday, Thursday, Saturday, and Sunday, but restrict calories on Tuesday and Friday. You choose the days of the week you fast, but you must incorporate a nonfasting day in between your fasting days.

What "normal" eating is for you depends on your height, weight, sex, and activity levels, as well as your weight goals. There are several free online calculators (you can search "online calorie calculator" to find many options) that let you type in your statistics and goals and get a recommendation on how many calories you should be eating on your "normal" days.

One study published in *International Journal of Obesity* monitored one hundred overweight females who were instructed to follow a Mediterranean-style diet for five days per week, while intermittent fasting (and only eating lean protein and few carbohydrates) on the other two days per week. When the study was concluded, the participants had lost significantly more weight than others who had focused on restricting calories for the entire week. Researchers also found that participants had better insulin sensitivity and a greater reduction in total body fat.

A separate study, published by researchers from the University of Florida and Harvard Medical School, found that following a 5:2 method of intermittent fasting can help control the stress response system, reducing stress and anxiety and thus improving the health of the nervous system. Researchers speculate that the combination of fasting and calorie restriction affects metabolism and cellular pathways in a positive way, protecting the nerve cells from negative genetic factors or environmental influences that cause aging of the cells.

Research also shows that the 5:2 method has a great success rate, even for those who have difficulty maintaining a normal daily diet routine. Once dieters adjust to the intermittent fasting plan, they tend to consume less food—and fewer calories—overall.

Alternate Day Fasting

There are two ways to do alternate day fasting. The first—and less common—way is to alternate days of eating normally with days of complete fasting. This means that you would eat normally on Monday, completely abstain from food Tuesday, eat normally on Wednesday, completely abstain from food on Thursday, and so on. The second way involves modified fasting. When you follow the modified alternative day fasting, you eat normally every other day and eat approximately one-fifth of your normal calories on the remaining days. For a typical diet of 2,000–2,500 calories per day, this means that you would eat 400–500 calories on your modified fasting days. The goal is to cut calories by 20–35 percent per week. Research shows that people are able to stick with alternate day fasting much easier than traditional low-calorie diets that require calorie restriction on every day of the week.

Like many of the other methods of fasting, you're allowed to drink as many calorie-free beverages as you want during your fasting time. If you choose to follow the modified fasting version, there are no restrictions about what times you consume your calories during the day. You can have one large meal during the day or spread mini meals or snacks out throughout the entire day.

Although alternate day fasting has been shown to reduce the risk of both type 2 diabetes and heart disease, this method of fasting was designed with weight loss in mind. According to studies involving overweight and obese adults, alternate day fasting may result in a 3–8 percent reduction in body weight in just two to twelve weeks; and unlike calorie restriction alone, alternate day fasting is shown to result in greater fat loss, especially abdominal fat, while preserving muscle mass. Combining alternate day fasting with endurance exercise, like running or swimming, can double the amount of weight lost; and according to one study published in *Obesity*, the combination of alternate day fasting and endurance exercise can help you lose up to six times as much weight as endurance exercise on its own.

Spontaneous Fasting

Unlike the other types of fasting, which are more rigid in their specific time frames, spontaneous fasting involves skipping meals spontaneously. For example, if you're not hungry in the morning, skip breakfast and eat only lunch and dinner. Or, if you're too busy to eat lunch, skip it.

The key with spontaneous fasting, though, is in making sure that you're eating healthy foods for the meals that you don't skip. Of course, this is important with all types of fasting, but it can be especially important with spontaneous fasting since there's less structure and the temptation to over-eat unhealthy foods may be higher.

Spontaneous fasting is a good way to get your feet wet with intermittent fasting. You can skip a meal here or there to get your body used to going an extended period of time without eating, then slowly transition to one of the other fasting plans. Or, if it works for you, you can stick with the spontaneous fasting indefinitely. Another benefit to spontaneous fasting is that it's easy to fit into your schedule because you can skip meals when it's convenient for you and eat meals when you have time to prepare something healthy.

Extended Fasting

Although extended fasting belongs to a class of its own, it's important to know the difference between it and the other types of intermittent fasting. Extended fasting is any type of fast that lasts for more than twenty-four hours. Often, extended fasting can last a week, and many of these extended fasts involve consuming only water.

These types of fasts are more common in medical and hospital settings and are usually done when the body needs to undergo significant healing or when the ability to eat is compromised. You should not start an extended fast without the recommendation and supervision of a medical professional.

Other Ways to Increase Autophagy

Although fasting is the most effective way to stimulate autophagy, you can also kick on this process through exercise and by following a ketogenic diet. This is why many people who fast decide to follow a ketogenic diet as well: it's a double whammy for cellular cleansing. The ketogenic diet helps stimulate autophagy by tricking the body into thinking it's going without food, so the same metabolic changes are seen. When you drastically lower carbohydrates, it forces your body to turn to using fat as an energy source instead. Doing this also keeps insulin levels low and glucagon levels high—a must for getting autophagy started.

Exercise is another effective way to stimulate autophagy, and because of this, regular exercise has been shown to kill cancerous cells. One study published in *Autophagy*, found that autophagy increases significantly after jogging for thirty minutes on a treadmill and continues increasing up to eighty total minutes of exercise, when it begins to level out. The effect is seen to a greater degree with intense exercise.

Choosing the Best Fasting Protocol for You

There are many different variations for intermittent fasting because there is no "one size fits all" approach. The plan that works best for you may not be the plan that works best for your neighbor, and vice versa. To decide which intermittent fasting type is best for you, you'll have to ask yourself a series of questions.

What's My Schedule Like?

One of the most important things to do is figure out which type of plan works best with your schedule. Of course, it's possible to rearrange your schedule around your new eating plan—and for some people this may be necessary—but you're more likely to stick to a new routine if it falls somewhat easily into your life. For many people, the 16/8 method is the plan that makes most sense with their schedule because most of the fasting time occurs overnight. However, if you're not on a typical schedule or you have longer work hours and you have to be up and ready to go for a longer portion of the day, this may not work as well for you. For example, if you don't work a typical Monday through Friday job and you have Monday and Thursday off instead, you may find that the 5:2 method works better for your schedule because you can eat normally while you're at work and then use your days off for your fasting days.

What Plan Will I Actually Stick To?

Sometimes, just figuring out which plan works best with your schedule isn't enough. In order to experience any lasting benefits of intermittent fasting, you'll have to actually stick to it. That being said, you'll need to find a plan that fits into your schedule. If the 16/8 method seems best in theory but you know you would have a hard time going for sixteen hours without food, then maybe a modified alternate day fasting protocol is better for you.

Make It Your Own

Don't put too much pressure on yourself to be perfect or to follow a certain protocol down to the letter, especially at first. Adjusting to intermittent fasting can take some time, especially if you're used to eating small meals all day long. Be gentle with yourself and give yourself time to adapt and adjust.

You can use the outlined methods to create your own protocol, or even mix up the protocols as you go. For example, you can follow the basics of the 16/8 method, but fast for thirteen to fourteen hours instead of sixteen.

You can use Eat Stop Eat as a template, but fast for sixteen or eighteen hours for a couple days each week until you can work your way up to a twenty-four-hour fast. Remember, the only way any of these methods will work is if you're able to stick to them. Modifying one of the protocols so that you can stick to it for the long haul is better than trying to follow a protocol exactly as written and quitting after a couple of weeks because you're so frustrated.

CHAPTER 5

What Do I Eat?

Nutrition is not a "one size fits all" process. Just as a tailor-made wardrobe would fit you best, a tailor-made nutrition plan will work best for you. That being said, there are some general nutrition concepts that you can use to figure out which foods work for you and which ones don't. While the main goal of fasting is to go for an extended period of time without eating, it's also important to eat healthy foods during your feeding windows. This will ensure that you're meeting your nutrition needs and feeding your body all the nutrients it needs to stay healthy and energized.

Choosing a Diet That's Right for You

Although the term *diet* is commonly associated with some type of food restriction, keep in mind that the real definition of *diet* is "the type of food a person habitually eats," and that's how you should interpret the term here. There's no specific diet that you must follow when intermittent fasting, but of course you'll reap the most benefits if you choose a diet full of nutrient-rich, unprocessed foods. There are some diets that are popular complements to intermittent fasting, but don't get caught up in dogma. You don't have to follow a diet plan exactly as written. For example, if you decide to follow a Paleo template but discover that your body does well with brown rice, you can add it in. You don't have to omit a food for good just because it doesn't fall under a dietary title. Use intuitive eating to figure out your best approach.

Ketogenic Diet

The ketogenic diet is one of the most popular diet companions to intermittent fasting. People who love intermittent fasting tend to lean toward this diet because the two approaches complement each other nicely: when used in combination, they'll quickly kick you into a chronic state of ketosis (a physiological state in which your body burns fat for energy instead of carbohydrates).

When following a ketogenic diet, most of your calories will come from fat, and your carbohydrate intake will be severely restricted. Unlike other diets, a ketogenic diet requires you to keep track of exactly how much fat, carbohydrates, and protein you're eating.

A typical ketogenic diet has a macronutrient breakdown as follows:

- 60–75 percent of calories from fat
- 15–30 percent of calories from protein
- 5–10 percent of calories from carbohydrates

Low-Carb Diet

A low-carb diet is similar to a ketogenic diet in that you restrict the amount of carbohydrates you take in each day. However, a traditional low-carb diet is not as high in fat and allows a more moderate intake of protein than a ketogenic diet does. Many low-carb diets suggest an initial period of very low-carbohydrate intake—around two weeks—where you remove almost all carbohydrate-containing foods, except low-carb vegetables. During this initial period, you'll lose a significant amount of water weight. After these two weeks, you'll move on to a more sustainable program in which you can include healthy sources of carbohydrates, such as other vegetables, some fruits, and gluten-free whole grains. The major goal of a standard low-carbohydrate diet is to lower blood sugar and insulin levels and promote weight loss.

Paleo Diet

The Paleo Diet is another popular companion to intermittent fasting because, like fasting, it's designed from the eating habits of your ancestors. The basic concept of a Paleo Diet is to consume only foods that were available to hunters and gatherers during the Paleolithic era. Of course, this definition is open to interpretation because your Paleolithic ancestors wouldn't have access to things like jars of almond butter, but you get the idea.

When following a Paleo Diet, you can eat:

- Meat
- Fish
- Poultry
- Eggs
- Nuts and seeds
- Fruits
- Healthy fats (avocado oil, coconut oil, olive oil, ghee)
- Natural sweeteners (raw honey, maple syrup, coconut sugar)

On the other hand, you'll need to avoid:

- Grains (wheat, oats, barley, rye, quinoa, couscous, amaranth, millet, corn)
- Dairy (milk, cheese, ice cream, butter)
- Legumes (soy, peanuts, chickpeas, beans)

- Alcohol
- Refined and artificial sweeteners (white sugar, high-fructose corn syrup, sucralose, aspartame)

There's a lot of debate about whether corn is classified as a vegetable or a grain. Technically, corn is considered a whole grain, and that's why it's excluded from the Paleo Diet. In addition to that, much of the corn grown in the United States is from GMO (genetically modified organism) crops, which Paleo Diet advocates try to steer clear of.

Pegan Diet

The Pegan Diet is a fairly new concept that was developed by Dr. Mark Hyman, the director of the Cleveland Clinic's Center for Functional Medicine. The Pegan diet combines the basic principles of the Paleo Diet and a vegan diet, which seems counterintuitive, since at first glance the diets appear to be on completely opposite ends of the spectrum; however, their basic principles are actually very similar.

Both the Paleo Diet and a vegan diet emphasize choosing whole, unprocessed foods that are responsibly sourced from the land. The major differences are that the Paleo Diet focuses on ethically sourced meats, vegetables, healthy fats, and some fruits, and eliminates all grains and legumes; a vegan diet eliminates all animal products and emphasizes grains, legumes, vegetables, and all plant-based foods. The goal of the Pegan diet is to combine the best things from the two diets.

When following the Pegan diet, plant-based foods will make up about 75 percent of your daily intake. You'll want to eat mostly vegetables; some fruits; some gluten-free grains, like quinoa, brown rice, and gluten-free oats; and some legumes, like lentils. The other 25 percent of your food intake should be in the form of high-quality animal proteins (grass-fed beef, pasture-raised chicken, and eggs) and healthy fats like coconut, olives, and avocados (and their respective oils: coconut oil, olive oil, and avocado oil). Dr. Hyman recommends treating meat more like a condiment than the main course. Instead of a typical 4–6-ounce serving, stick to 2–3 ounces of meat per meal.

While following a Pegan diet, you'll avoid gluten, dairy, and some vegetable oils (canola, sunflower, corn, and soybean). Sugar—even natural types like honey and maple syrup—should be eaten only as an occasional treat. Although natural sugars do provide some health benefits, overdoing them can negatively affect blood sugar levels—something you're ultimately trying to avoid when intermittent fasting.

Low-FODMAP Diet

FODMAPs, which stands for fermentable oligosaccharides, disaccharides, monosaccharides, and polyols, are short-chain carbohydrates that can cause digestive distress in those who have digestive sensitivities. A low-FODMAP diet is typically recommended for someone who is experiencing chronic digestive trouble or unexplained irritable bowel syndrome. When following a low-FODMAP diet, you'll avoid certain categories of carbohydrates, which include:

- Oligosaccharides: wheat, rye, legumes, garlic, onions, leeks, asparagus, jicama, fennel, beetroot, and Brussels sprouts
- Disaccharides: white sugar, milk, yogurt, and soft cheeses like cream cheese and cottage cheese
- Monosaccharides: peaches, plums, pears, nectarines, mangoes, watermelon, apples, and honey
- Polyols: blackberries, avocados, sweet potatoes, cauliflower, snow peas, and mushrooms

When following a low-FODMAP diet, you'll completely eliminate all high-FODMAP foods for about one month. After this initial elimination period, you can reintroduce one high-FODMAP food at a time to see how your body reacts. If you don't experience any digestive upset, it's likely your body can handle that food. If you do, it's likely that you're sensitive to it and you'd do well to avoid it as much as possible.

Basic Nutrition Elements

Of course, it's not necessary to box yourself into a certain dietary principle. You can use basic nutrition concepts (like eating only fresh, whole foods, avoiding processed foods and sugar, and eating plenty of fruits and vegetables) to experiment with different types of foods and determine which foods work for you and which foods you should avoid.

Grains

Grains are quite the hot topic. It seems that nutrition experts—and the general population—are divided down the middle when it comes to whether grains are good or bad for you. One side of the debate recommends avoiding grains, while the other side says that whole grains are a necessity due to their fiber and vitamin B content. So, who is right? Well, the answer is that it depends. The anti-grains side says that there are three major problems with grains: lectins, phytates, and gluten.

Lectins

Lectins are a type of protein found in both grains and legumes and bind to cell membranes. They are small and hard to digest because they're resistant to both heat and digestive enzymes. Because of this, they tend to accumulate in your body and travel into your blood in their whole form. When proteins enter your blood whole, your immune system develops antibodies, which means that it recognizes the protein as a foreign invader and builds up an attack system against it. Over time this can result in leaky gut and increased sensitivity to lectins.

Lectins serve as a defense mechanism for a plant. They are meant to keep pests, insects, and microorganisms from eating (and destroying) the plant. Because lectins are resistant to digestion, they pass through the digestive system unchanged, so the plant can regrow once excreted.

Phytates

Phytates are compounds found in grains and legumes and in lesser amounts in nuts and seeds. Phytates are not inherently bad for you, but they're often described as antinutrients because they bind to minerals like iron, zinc, and calcium, preventing their absorption. This can set you up for mineral deficiencies. It's important to note here that phytates don't impair your ability to absorb nutrients over the long term; they only block absorption during that meal.

Gluten

Of course, when it comes to grains, gluten is the most controversial. While celiac disease—an inability to properly digest gluten—is widely accepted, many people don't believe in non-celiac gluten sensitivity. But research shows that gluten can damage the intestinal lining (and cause celiac disease symptoms), even in people who don't have the disease.

Scientists from the University of Maryland discovered that when you eat gluten, your body produces a protein called zonulin. Zonulin negatively affects the gut lining by creating spaces between the intestinal cells, which are normally extremely tight. When these spaces are created, food and microbes are able to pass through them and enter the blood. Once in the blood, these particles trigger an immune response that never gets shut off. This response can cause inflammation and, eventually, chronic disease. It's also the underlying factor of many autoimmune diseases. This is called "leaky gut" and recent evidence shows that people who consume gluten have at least a mild form of it.

A Note on Wheat

Wheat has been a part of agriculture for over nine thousand years and is one of the largest crops in the world. It's considered an integral part of many nations' food supply because it can be stored in kernel form for years and can be processed to make a wide variety of foods, including flour, breads, noodles, and cereals. The problem with wheat is not in the grain itself, but what modern agriculture has done to it.

The wheat of today is not only lower in many nutrients that were in wheat of the past, but the structure of the plant itself has been changed due to modern milling. The goal of modern processes is to create a crop that can survive should disaster strike, so major food corporations have made it resistant to drought, adverse weather, pests, and chemicals. As a result of this, your body doesn't recognize wheat the way that it used to. Instead of providing nourishment, it's become inflammatory and addictive.

Making Grains Healthier

If you want to include grains in your diet, there are a few things you can do to ensure that your body tolerates them better. First, choose gluten-free grains. It's estimated that around 1 percent of the population suffers from celiac disease, while up to 13 percent have non-celiac gluten sensitivity. Signs of gluten sensitivity include:

- Bloating
- Constipation and/or diarrhea
- Abdominal pain
- Headaches
- Fatigue
- Skin problems (rashes, psoriasis, eczema, hives, dermatitis)
- Depression
- Unexplained weight loss
- Iron-deficiency anemia
- Anxiety
- Joint or muscle pain
- Autoimmune disorders
- Brain fog

Gluten-free grains include brown rice, wild rice, quinoa, buckwheat, millet, teff, and amaranth. Oats are technically gluten-free as well, but because of the way they're manufactured, they're almost always contaminated by gluten. If you want to include oats in your diet, choose brands that are specifically labeled as gluten-free.

The next thing you can do is soak your grains before consumption. Soaking grains can help break down the phytates and neutralize the lectins, so the grains are easier to digest and you are able to absorb all of the minerals in them. To soak the grains, place them in a bowl and cover completely with warm, filtered water. For every cup of water you add to the bowl, you must also add one tablespoon of an acidic medium, such as lemon juice or apple cider vinegar. For example, if you need three cups of water to cover your grains, add three tablespoons of lemon juice to the water, then cover the bowl with a breathable medium, like a clean kitchen towel. Next, let the grains sit for twelve hours. After the grains have soaked for an adequate amount of time, rinse them off with cold water and proceed with your recipe as usual.

Another option is to sprout your grains or to use grains that have already been sprouted. Food manufacturers have caught on to the health benefits of sprouting your grains, and many companies now offer grains that are already sprouted, which can save you time and effort. If you can't find already sprouted grains in your local grocery store, you can look online or sprout them yourself.

Because brown rice has lower phytate levels than some of the other gluten-free grains, it only takes about seven hours of soaking time to break them down.

Sprouting takes considerably longer than soaking grains because you have to wait for the grain to actually crack open and form a sprout. To sprout your own grains, follow the process for soaking and then transfer the soaked and drained grains to a glass jar—a Mason jar works well. Cover the jar with a cheesecloth and allow the grains to sit in the moist jar for one to five days. You'll know when they're ready because the grains will crack open and a green sprout will be visible. You can store sprouted grains in the refrigerator for up to one week.

Dairy

Dairy is another controversial product in the nutrition world. You probably grew up hearing about how great milk is for your bones. The truth is that milk is not as good for your bones as you may think. In fact, the countries with the lowest milk consumption have the lowest rates of fractures and osteoporosis, a condition in which the bones become brittle and are more prone to breaks and fractures. In addition, many people have trouble digesting the proteins and sugars found in milk. This is because as you age, your body's production of lactase—the enzyme that you need to digest milk properly—naturally decreases.

However, this doesn't mean that you can't consume any dairy, but there are some options that are better than others. If you are going to include dairy in your diet, choose dairy that comes from grass-fed cows. You can usually find grass-fed milk, butter, and cheese at local stores. Grass-fed dairy has a higher content of omega-3s, unlike conventional dairy, which has more omega-6s. Omega-6s aren't inherently bad, but when you eat too many (which many Americans do), it can lead to chronic inflammation. Cultured grass-fed dairy products, like yogurt and kefir, are also good choices; however, make sure they are full-fat and plain. Flavored yogurts and kefirs are often loaded with sugar.

If you want to avoid cow's milk completely, goat's milk products are a great option. Modern cow's milk contains high amounts of a protein called A1 casein, which can be very inflammatory (and cause issues like eczema and acne). On the other hand, goat's milk contains a protein called A2 casein, which is not inflammatory. Studies show that people who consume milk with A2 casein experienced reduced inflammation and no negative digestive symptoms.

Meat and Poultry

Meat is another controversial product that has been vilified over the years due to its saturated-fat content. When low-fat diets became really popular, red meat was a major no-no; but since then, science has shown that saturated fat doesn't have as great an impact on heart disease as previously thought. In fact, the right types of saturated fat can protect against heart disease.

The old school of thought was that saturated fat raised cholesterol, which increased the risk of heart disease; but research now shows that while saturated fats can raise the amount of LDL in your blood, it creates the large, fluffy LDL particles that don't stick to the artery walls. Saturated fat also raises HDL levels, which is what protects against heart disease.

Meat is also one of the top sources of vitamin B_{12}. In fact, you can only get vitamin B_{12} from animal products. Meat also contains the other B vitamins, vitamin D, vitamin E, amino acids, antioxidants, and several minerals.

That being said, just like with dairy, it's important to choose high-quality, grass-fed meats. Conventional meat comes from cows that are fed GMO crops, grains, and even sugar. This fattens the cows up more quickly so they produce more, but it also affects the nutritional content of their meat.

Grass-fed meat also contains up to five times more omega-3 fatty acids than conventional meat and significantly fewer omega-6s.

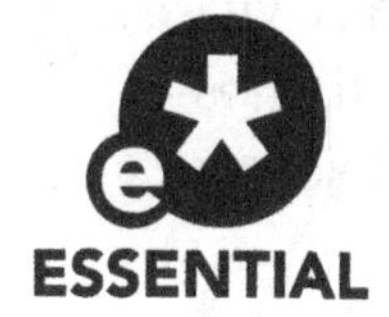

To keep inflammation at bay, you want to aim for a 1:1 ratio of omega-3 fatty acids to omega 6 fatty acids. Many of the foods available today, like conventional meat and refined seed and vegetable oils, are high in omega-6 fatty acids. Eating too many of these foods can throw off this ratio, which promotes chronic inflammation in your body.

Grass-fed meat also contains a fat called conjugated linoleic acid, or CLA. CLA acts as an antioxidant and has been shown to reduce the risk of heart disease, stop the growth of cancerous tumors, prevent atherosclerosis, decrease triglycerides, and reduce the risk of developing type 2 diabetes. All animal foods contain some amount of CLA, but grass-fed meat and dairy contain up to 500 percent more than dairy and meat that comes from grain-fed cows.

As with meat, not all poultry is the same. There is poultry that comes from conventional farms, and then there is poultry that's raised organically and allowed to roam freely, eating a natural diet. Often you'll see labels on poultry and eggs that boast that the birds were "fed a vegetarian diet," but chickens and turkeys are not vegetarians. They like to scavenge for bugs, ticks, and worms, and that is what makes the chicken so nutritious. Poultry that has been allowed to consume a natural diet is higher in omega-3s, vitamins, and minerals.

When choosing poultry, it's best to choose a combination of organic and pasture raised. If this is unavailable at your local grocery store or your budget doesn't allow for it, talk to your local farmers. Often you may find high-quality meats at your local farms that aren't labeled pasture raised or organic (because these are government-moderated terms, and many small farms can't afford to pay for the certification process required to carry these labels) but by definition are both of these things.

A Note on Eggs

There is a lot of fear surrounding cholesterol, so people often separate their eggs, throwing away the yolk and eating only the egg white. While the white of the egg contains protein, most of the nutrients, like vitamin A, vitamin D, vitamin E, vitamin K, B vitamins, omega-3 fats, calcium, and phosphorus in an egg are found in its yolk. Don't be scared to eat the whole egg, but do choose the types of eggs you consume wisely.

Many of the labels and nutritional claims on eggs are just marketing tactics. For example, the terms *natural* and *farm fresh* usually mean nothing. Other terms, like *cage-free*, sound good, but they can be misleading. When you hear the term *cage-free*, you may picture birds roaming around outside in the sunlight, but *cage-free* just means that the birds were not in cages. They could still have been in an overcrowded warehouse without much room to move. The best type of eggs you can get are organic and pasture raised. Again, talking to your local egg farmers is a great way to find high-quality eggs that are usually fresher and less expensive than the eggs you'll find in a grocery store.

Seafood

Seafood is loaded with protein and beneficial vitamins and minerals, but the most notable health benefits tied to seafood come from two specific omega-3 fatty acids: eicosapentaenoic acid (EPA) and docosahexaenoic acid (DHA). Regular consumption of EPA and DHA has been shown to reduce the risk of heart disease, cancer, type 2 diabetes, and autoimmune diseases.

When choosing fish, it's best to consume smaller species of fish. Larger fish that are higher on the food chain tend to accumulate more mercury and other heavy metals and toxins in their flesh.

The fish and shellfish that are highest in omega-3s include:

- Salmon
- Mackerel
- Trout
- Sardines
- Herring
- Oysters
- Mussels

Tuna and swordfish are also rich in omega-3s, but they are contaminated with mercury. If you choose tuna and swordfish, limit consumption. There is one company, called Safe Catch, that offers safer canned tuna with the lowest possible levels of mercury.

In addition to choosing smaller fish that are high in omega-3 fatty acids, it's also best to choose fish that have been wild caught rather than farm raised. As with animals that are raised for conventional meat, farmed fish is fed a diet that is not natural to them. This may include corn and grains. As a result of their unnatural diet, farm-raised fish become high in omega-6 fatty acids and lower in omega-3 fatty acids. In fact, according to one analysis published in the *Journal of the American Dietetic Association*, omega-3 fatty acids couldn't even be detected in some farm-raised fish found in grocery stores. In addition to the altered levels of fatty acids, farm-raised fish accumulate higher levels of toxins and contaminants in their flesh.

Fruits and Vegetables

You know that fruits and vegetables are good for you. Of course, some fruit contains more natural sugar than others, but when this sugar is combined with the fiber in the fruit, it's not a problem for most people. Problems arise from drinking too much fruit juice, which contains all of the sugar without any of the fiber, so when eating fruit, make sure to eat it whole and ideally with the skin on (which contains fiber).

There's also research that shows that organic produce not only contains fewer pesticides and herbicides than conventional produce, but that it is also richer in some vitamins and minerals. If your budget doesn't allow for a lot of organic choices, you can prioritize which fruits and vegetables to purchase organic by using the Environmental Working Group's Dirty Dozen list. The Dirty Dozen list outlines which fruits and vegetables typically have the most contamination. These are the produce items that you should prioritize buying organic. The Dirty Dozen are:

- Strawberries
- Spinach
- Nectarines
- Apples
- Grapes
- Peaches
- Cherries
- Pears
- Tomatoes
- Celery
- Potatoes
- Sweet bell peppers

In addition to the Dirty Dozen list, the Environmental Working Group also supplies a list of the produce that tends to contain the lowest amount of pesticides and contaminants. These fruits and vegetables are the ones that you don't have to prioritize buying organic. This list is called the Clean Fifteen and they are:

- Avocados
- Sweet corn
- Pineapples
- Cabbage
- Onions
- Frozen sweet peas
- Papayas
- Asparagus
- Mangos
- Eggplant
- Honeydew melons
- Kiwis
- Cantaloupes
- Cauliflower
- Broccoli

Fats and Oils

Fat is nothing to fear. In fact, including healthy fats in your diet can provide valuable vitamins and minerals and help keep you full longer. The key is to choose fats that are good for you. Natural, healthy fats are vital components of a balanced diet.

Margarine contains trans fats in the form of hydrogenated oils. Trans fats were created to give foods a longer shelf life, but they have a detrimental effect on cholesterol levels. Unlike saturated fats, which increase the large, fluffy LDL particles that don't stick to the artery walls, trans fats increase the small, dense LDL particles that get stuck on the artery walls and can cause blockages that increase your risk for heart disease.

The FDA has a list of food ingredients, called "generally recognized as safe" (GRAS), that they claim are safe for human consumption. In 2015, the FDA removed trans fats from the list and required food manufacturers to start removing any ingredients that contain trans fats from their products.

Refined oils, like soybean oil, which is a common ingredient in many prepackaged foods, are high in omega-6 fatty acids. As you've already learned, eating too many omega-6 fatty acids can contribute to chronic inflammation, which is connected to a number of diseases and health issues.

The best fats to consume include:

- Olive oil
- Avocado oil
- Unsalted grass-fed butter
- Grass-fed ghee
- Coconut oil
- Walnut oil
- Hemp oil
- Sesame oil

Cooking with Fats

All fats have a certain smoke point (a point at which they start to smoke when exposed to a certain temperature). When fats reach their smoke point, the process can break down some of the antioxidants and vitamins and even create compounds that are harmful to your health. You should use care to only cook with oils that have a high smoke point, especially when you're using high heat. Avocado oil, butter, ghee, and coconut oil all have the highest smoke points and are the best for cooking. Olive oil can be used for cooking, but only on low heat. Walnut oil, hemp oil, and sesame oil are best used as dressings or eaten cool.

It's also best to store fats away from a heat source. If you store your fats next to the stove, the residual heat from cooking can make them go rancid.

Sugar and Sweeteners

Most of the health problems that are often blamed on fat are really due to sugar. Sugar doesn't have any health benefits, yet the average American consumes approximately 66 pounds of sugar per year. Even more concerning than having no nutritional value is the fact that sugar contributes to chronic inflammation, increases your risk of heart disease, destabilizes blood sugar levels, and feeds cancer cells. Eating too much sugar can also make it easy for you to gain weight.

Manufacturers have tried to solve the problem of sugar by introducing artificial sweeteners to the market, but studies show that people who consume artificial sweeteners have a greater risk of diabetes, metabolic syndrome, and heart disease. Artificial sweeteners can also throw off the balance of bacteria in your gut, causing both digestive and systemic issues. Artificial sweeteners have also been linked to cancer and chronic migraines. In addition to that, when you give your body the sweet taste without any calories, it can lead to sugar cravings that are even more intense.

No matter what form it's in, sugar should be limited as much as possible. However, there are certain sweeteners that are better for you than others. The best choices include:

- Pure maple syrup
- Raw honey
- Coconut sugar
- Date sugar

- Monk fruit
- Molasses
- Stevia
- Erythritol

A Note on Stevia

Although stevia is a plant and is marketed as natural, many packaged forms are highly processed by the time they're available to you. In addition to that, some stevia products also contain added ingredients, like "natural flavors," that are unfavorable. The term "natural flavors" is not closely regulated by the FDA, and companies are free to use this description even for chemical additives that mimic natural flavors. If you choose to use stevia, do so sparingly and make sure you're choosing one that's pure and organic.

CHAPTER 6

Fasting Myths and Questions

There are many misconceptions surrounding intermittent fasting. Of course, it's normal for people who don't understand how fasting works to question whether purposely going without food really is good for you. The following are answers to some of the most commonly asked questions and the most persistent myths about intermittent fasting.

Will Starvation Mode Kick In?

Starvation mode is one of the most common concerns of people who are new to intermittent fasting. To be clear, starvation mode (adaptive thermogenesis) is a real thing; however, how it works is often misunderstood.

When you eat food, your body either uses it for any immediate energy needs or stores it in fat tissue for later use. If a greater number of calories enter the fat tissue than the number of calories that leave it, you gain fat. If the opposite happens, you lose fat. This is the basis of the "calories in, calories out" theory (although the science is becoming more and more clear that not all calories are created equal). When you're trying to lose weight, you typically restrict calories in some way. This prompts an imbalance between calories in and calories out that will likely allow you to lose weight. You see this as a good thing, but your body sees it as a bad thing.

Your body's main concern is survival, and when you start to burn off extra calories and lose fat in the process, your body sees it as a threat—the beginning of an impending starvation. As a result, in an effort to save itself, your body starts to conserve calories and doesn't burn them off as effectively, so over time—and after significant weight loss—your calorie needs go down. This is adaptive thermogenesis.

What is norepinephrine?
Norepinephrine, also called noradrenaline, belongs to a family of body chemicals called catecholamines. It's released into the blood by the sympathetic nervous system in response to anything that the brain perceives as a stressful event. The release of norepinephrine increases heart rate, triggers the release of glucose into the blood, increases blood flow, and speeds up reaction time. The neurotransmitter is a vital component of the body's fight-or-flight response.

Many people believe that the solution to keeping your body from going into starvation mode is to eat small meals frequently. That's why you hear the advice that it's better to eat five or six small meals throughout the day than to eat two or three larger meals. However, while adaptive thermogenesis is a real thing, it doesn't quite work like that. The only way your body will enter a true starvation mode is if you go a prolonged period of time—days or weeks, as opposed to hours—without eating. If the body went into starvation mode within hours, it would be highly disadvantageous to the survival of the human species. In Paleolithic times, a decrease in metabolism would also mean a decrease in energy, which would make it harder to hunt and gather food. If hunters and gatherers couldn't obtain food, metabolism would drop even more and energy would continue to plummet, eventually leading to an inability to survive.

Studies show that intermittent fasting doesn't inhibit your ability to burn off extra calories and fat: it actually has the opposite effect on your metabolic rate. According to research published in *The American Journal of Clinical Nutrition* and *The American Journal of Physiology*, the number of calories you burn at rest—also called your basal metabolic rate (or BMR)—actually increases by a significant amount when you incorporate short-term fasting. The reason for this is that when you enter a fasted state, the levels of norepinephrine—a stress hormone and neurotransmitter—in your blood decrease. This stimulates your metabolism and signals your body to break down excess body fat.

Don't You Lose Muscle by Fasting?

It's a common belief that if you miss a meal your body will immediately start turning to your muscles as an energy source, but thanks to human evolution it doesn't work like that.

In order for the body to achieve its main goal of survival, it has to obtain energy. Its preferred source is glucose, which comes mainly from carbohydrates. If glucose is not available, the body will then turn to body fat, which is essentially stored energy. Remember: when you eat an excess of calories, your body converts them to triglycerides and stores those triglycerides in your fat cells. The body instinctively knows to use muscle as an energy source only when glucose and body fat are too low to sustain life. This only happens when body fat dips below 4 percent, which is extremely low. To put it into perspective, male athletes typically have a body fat percentage of 6–13 percent, while female athletes have around 14–20 percent. Your body will preserve muscle mass until body fat becomes so low that it has no choice but to use protein for fuel. Most people never reach this point.

It's true that when you restrict calories without incorporating any form of resistance training, there's a possibility that you'll lose some muscle mass; but fasting doesn't increase the amount of muscle mass that you lose. In fact, research shows that people who incorporate fasting into their weight-loss plan experience less of a reduction in lean muscle mass than those who don't intermittently fast.

Will My Blood Sugar Get Too Low?

One of the most common concerns when it comes to intermittent fasting centers around blood sugar. At some point in your life, you've probably experienced the symptoms of low blood sugar—hunger, irritability, weakness, sweaty palms, or anxiety—when you've gone too long without eating. While it's true that low blood sugar can be unpleasant, it's not the fact that you've gone without eating that causes your blood sugar to dip too low: it's what you ate during your previous meal.

When you eat a meal that's loaded with carbohydrates, it sends a rush of glucose into your bloodstream. Your body responds to the glucose rush by releasing insulin to carry it into the cells so you can use it as energy. The higher your glucose spikes, the more insulin that's sent out; the more insulin that's sent out, the more your blood sugar ultimately drops over time. When you combine fasting with a healthy, moderate- to low-carbohydrate diet, your body is extremely efficient in managing blood glucose levels on its own, so you don't experience those dramatic spikes and dips in your blood sugar even when you go for an extended period of time without eating.

If you have problems with blood sugar control or if you're diabetic, the glucose and insulin response doesn't work as well, so make sure to speak with your healthcare provider before starting any type of fast to determine if it's right for you.

Does Fasting Lead to Binges?

There's a popular belief that if you go too long without eating, you'll end up binging on unhealthy foods once you do eat, ultimately gaining weight. It's not so black and white: there are many factors to consider.

Studies on alternate day fasting show that people who fast tend to take in more calories on the day after a twenty-four-hour fast, however, the increase is under 500 calories. So, if you factor the calories missed during fasting into the minimal increase in intake the next day, it still comes out to a calorie deficit.

The desire to binge is often also caused by the dramatic dip in blood sugar that occurs after a carbohydrate-rich meal or due to a carbohydrate addiction. Once your blood sugar levels off after a period of time of intermittent fasting, you'll notice that hunger stabilizes and you have less of a desire to eat in excess.

For those who have struggled with bulimia or binge-eating disorder, it's possible that fasting can lead to binges or bulimic behavior. Make sure to speak with your healthcare provider before starting intermittent fasting if you have a history of disordered eating.

When Should I Exercise While Fasting?

There's a long-standing debate in the fitness world about whether it's better to work out on an empty stomach (a fasted state) or a full stomach (a fed state). The answer is that it depends on the intensity of your exercise. There are many benefits to exercising in a fasted state, but if you're an endurance athlete or engaging in high-intensity exercise, working out after eating may be better for you.

When you exercise, your body demands an increased amount of energy. First, your body will turn for fuel to glucose in the blood. When that runs out, it starts burning glycogen—the form of glucose that's stored in the liver. In general, your liver stores enough glycogen to sustain your body's energy needs for twenty-four hours in the absence of food; however, the increased energy demand that exercise puts on the body will result in a faster depletion of glycogen. The amount of glycogen that gets used up depends on the duration and the intensity of the exercise you're doing.

Once glycogen is depleted, your body switches from burning carbohydrates for energy to burning stored fat. Your body's ability to burn fat is controlled by your sympathetic nervous system, which is turned on by both fasting and exercise. When you combine the two, it maximizes the physiological processes that break down fat for energy. Unlike glycogen, which is only stored in limited amounts, fat can be stored in your body in unlimited amounts, so you never run out. Your muscles will eventually adapt to using whatever energy source you give them.

The term *hitting a wall*, or *"bonking,"* is used to describe the sudden fatigue and loss of energy that occurs when glycogen stores are fully depleted. This is common in endurance athletes—like marathon runners and triathletes.

One study published in the *International Journal of Sport Nutrition and Exercise Metabolism* placed nineteen men into each of two groups. The first group of men engaged in aerobic exercise (cardio) in a fasted state, while the second group of men did their cardio in a fed state. During each exercise session, the participants had their measurements taken, filled out a food questionnaire, and provided blood and urine samples. After the study was concluded, researchers discovered that while both groups of men experienced weight loss, only the men in the fasted group lowered their body-fat percentage. In other words, while the men in the fed group lost weight, they still had the same relative amount of body fat.

Fasting and exercise also put a good kind of stress on your body, which makes your muscles more resilient and helps counteract the effects of muscle aging. When this stress is put on your body, it triggers the release of brain-derived neurotrophic factor (BDNF) and muscle regulatory factors (MRFs), which send messages to the brain to create new neurons and which trigger the muscles to make new muscle cells.

This cascade of events does much more than help you lose fat or build muscle: the release of BDNF and MRFs, and the resulting creation of new neurons and muscles cells, can keep your brain, neurons, and muscle fibers biologically young, boost brain function, prevent depression, boost testosterone levels, and increase levels of growth hormone in the body.

Hormonal Benefits of Fasted Exercise

In addition to increasing fat burn, exercising on an empty stomach has also been shown to optimize health by improving levels of two specific hormones: insulin and growth hormone.

Research shows that fasted exercise may have a positive effect on insulin sensitivity (the way the body responds to insulin). When you eat too much, your blood sugar spikes, and as a result your body is exposed to a constant barrage of insulin. Over time this can cause an insulin overload that weakens the way your cells respond to the hormone. By exercising in a fasted state, you're not only giving your body a break from releasing insulin into the blood but you're also burning up any excess insulin that your body may have. When your body responds to insulin in a healthy way, it makes it easier to lose fat and improves blood flow to muscles, making them easier to build. Fasted exercise increases the production of growth hormone, which not only helps burn fat and increase muscle tissue but also improves bone health.

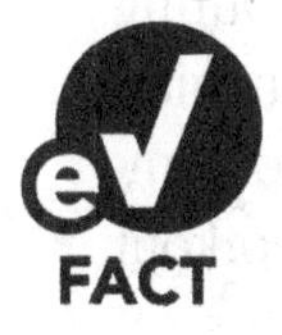

If you have diabetes, especially type 1 diabetes, please discuss any changes to your exercise routine with your healthcare provider. Exercising while fasted can drop both insulin and glucose levels, which can be dangerous for someone who is on diabetes medications or unable to properly regulate insulin levels.

It's also beneficial to wait at least sixty to ninety minutes before eating after a workout. Many people think that to maximize the results of a workout you have to eat a large amount of protein immediately afterward, but going an hour to an hour and a half without eating after working out actually maximizes fat loss because your metabolic rate is elevated post-exercise.

Tips for Exercise

Regular exercise is a vital component to staying healthy, so while it can take some extra planning to get into the proper groove when you're intermittent fasting, it's important that you keep a regular routine. Although it always comes back to listening to your body's specific needs, there are a few general tips to get you started in developing your plan.

Do Light-Intensity Exercise in a Fasted State

When you're in a fasted state, your body is depleted of glycogen, which means that you likely won't have the stamina to bust out high-intensity training.

If you're exercising while fasted, stick to lighter intensity exercises like walking, yoga, or elliptical training. Endurance exercise, like running for a couple of hours, may also make it more likely that your body will turn to protein for fuel, so stick to workouts that are an hour or shorter when you're fasting.

Do High-Intensity Exercise in a Fed State

On the days when you want to do high-intensity exercise, like HIIT (or High-Intensity Interval Training: a type of workout where you alternate short bursts of high-intensity exercise with longer periods of lower intensity exercise) or strength training, schedule your training close to a meal. When you exercise in a fed state, you provide your body with glucose and glycogen to push you through your workouts. This will prevent muscle loss as well as low blood sugar levels.

A good way to gauge the intensity of your workout is the talk test. During a low-intensity workout, you should be able to carry on a conversation fairly easily. When the exercise is high-intensity, you should only be able to comfortably say a few words at a time. If you can't talk at all during your workout without losing your breath, you're exercising too hard.

Timing Is Everything

If you're looking to build some serious muscle, schedule all strength-training sessions between two meals. Your muscles need amino acids to repair themselves and grow after weight lifting, so if adding muscle is your goal, eat a protein-rich meal an hour before your strength-training session, and another protein-rich meal sixty to ninety minutes after your workout is over. According to the Academy of Nutrition and Dietetics, you should aim for 20–30 grams of high-quality protein per meal.

Keep in mind that many people easily eat well over their recommended protein needs each day, so you don't have to go crazy. To give you some perspective, a 6-ounce chicken breast contains 52 grams of protein.

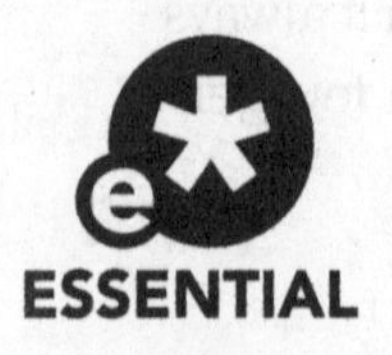

If you're concerned about losing muscle during your workout, you may want to consider supplementing branched-chain amino acids (BCAAs). Three branched-chain amino acids, leucine, isoleucine, and valine, comprise 35 percent of your muscle protein. Taking 5–10 grams of BCAAs as a supplement before training can help prevent muscle breakdown.

Now I Can Eat Whatever I Want, Right?

Many people who incorporate intermittent fasting follow a ketogenic diet or a Paleo-style dietary regimen, but that's not necessary for success. It's up to you to decide which style of eating works best for your body, and that may take some experimentation. The recipes in this book are all gluten-free, refined-sugar-free, and soy-free. As a general rule, the closer the food is to its natural state, the better.

The Importance of Micronutrients

Most of the major diets put an emphasis on macronutrients (carbohydrates, protein, and fat). There are low-carbohydrate, high-fat diets and low-fat, high-carbohydrate diets. There is also IIFYM, "if it fits your macros," which is based on the principle that you can eat whatever you want as long as you maintain the ratio of carbohydrates, proteins, and fats that is right for your body. Although some of these diets do focus on food quality, many of them are missing a major piece of the health puzzle: micronutrients.

Macronutrients are named for the fact that the body needs them in large amounts. Conversely, micronutrients are so-named because the body needs them in smaller amounts. Unlike micronutrients, macronutrients also provide the body with calories.

Carbohydrates, proteins, and fats are macronutrients; vitamins and minerals are micronutrients. However, just because the body needs micronutrients in smaller amounts, it doesn't mean they're less important. In fact, the importance of getting adequate amounts of micronutrients cannot be overstated.

All vitamins and minerals fall into the category of micronutrients. There are thirteen vitamins and sixteen minerals that you need adequate amounts of every single day to stay healthy. Each one of these vitamins and minerals performs crucial functions in the body to keep everything running smoothly. For example, vitamin C promotes collagen function, which is a critical component of your bones, joints, and skin. Vitamin D helps strengthen your bones and plays an important role in immune function. Sodium and potassium work together to control fluid and electrolyte balance. The B vitamins allow you to properly metabolize carbohydrates, proteins, and fats. Vitamin B_6 also supports the creation of new blood cells and neurotransmitters. Your body needs vitamin A in order to see colors and in dark lighting. Without vitamin K, your blood won't clot properly. Calcium helps your muscles contract and allows nerves to send signals to each other. Of course, this only touches the surface. There are countless other roles that these and other vitamins and minerals play. Magnesium alone is involved in over three hundred chemical reactions in the body!

If your intake of vitamins and minerals falls short, over time you'll develop a deficiency. Although it might not seem like a big issue, even a small deficiency in one micronutrient can cause major health problems. For example, low levels of vitamin D have been associated with depression (especially seasonal affective disorder, which occurs in the winter months) and irritable bowel syndrome. Magnesium deficiency can cause irregular heartbeat, muscle twitching and cramps, high blood pressure, fatigue, depression, and apathy (lack of emotion). Deficiencies in vitamin B_{12} can cause anemia, tingling in the hands and feet, fatigue, weakness, irritability, and depression. If a B_{12} deficiency becomes severe, it can present psychological conditions such as dementia, paranoia, and major depression.

These effects are alarming and can be quite devastating, and research shows that most people are deficient in at least one micronutrient. The United States Department of Agriculture (USDA) reports that most adult Americans don't get enough calcium, potassium, magnesium, vitamin A, vitamin C, vitamin D, and vitamin E in their daily diets. One study published in the *Journal of the International Society of Sports Nutrition* analyzed seventy different dietary intakes from a group of men and women and found that on average, males' diets were lacking in 40 percent of the vitamins and just over 54 percent of the minerals. The females' diets were slightly better but were still deficient in 29 percent of the vitamins and just over 44 percent of the minerals.

Although there are no strict rules on what to eat during your meals while intermittent fasting, the best way to get adequate amounts of each micronutrient and prevent micronutrient deficiencies is to eat a balanced diet that contains a wide variety of fruits and vegetables and limits nutrient-deficient foods like processed and packaged foods.

Eating Mindfully

A meal should be something that you savor, not something that you rush through at your desk while working or in your car between errands. Part of optimal health is eating slowly and mindfully so that you can enjoy every bite—and you can pay attention to signals that tell you when you've had enough. Since you'll be eating fewer meals when you're intermittent fasting, it's even more of a reason to slow down and enjoy the process.

Treat your meals like they're an important part of your day and not just an afterthought. When it's time to eat, stop everything else and sit down for a proper meal. Prepare your body for digestion by taking a deep breath and transitioning into a relaxed state.

Research shows that those who eat while distracted—like when sitting in front of the television—miss important cues from the body that signal satiety and as a result eat more than they would if they were eating without any distractions.

Mindful eating is a great way to learn how to listen to your body and practice balance. Here are a few tips to get you started:

1. Forget about Cleaning Your Plate. From a young age, you're taught to clear everything off of your plate. You may have been told not to waste food or that there are starving children in other parts of the world that would love a hot meal. While the sentiment behind those statements is meant to be positive, they can backfire in the long term. You carry those ideas into adulthood and may have a tendency to eat every bite of food on your plate, even if you're full halfway through the meal. This isn't to say you should waste food, but instead of overstuffing yourself in the interest of clearing your plate, serve yourself a smaller portion to begin with, or save what you can't eat for your next meal. Listen to your body and the signals that tell you you're full—and honor those signals.
2. Opt for Smaller Plates. It may be a trick of the mind, but smaller plates can help with portion control. When you're holding a plate, you tend to fill it. That means that when you have a large plate, you'll typically serve

yourself more food than if you had a smaller plate. Instead of a dinner plate, opt for a salad or appetizer plate. You can go always go back for seconds if you're still hungry, but give yourself some time to allow your food to settle.

3. Put Utensils Down Between Bites. Today's world is "go, go, go." People tend to rush through their entire days—and eating is no different. Next time you sit down for a meal, take a breath and slow down. Put your fork down between bites and chew slowly instead of rushing to get in and swallow each bite as quickly as you can.
4. Pay Attention. When was the last time you paid attention to the texture of the food you were eating? The crunch of almonds in your mouth, the tanginess of your salad dressing, and the coolness of a bite of avocado often go unnoticed when you're rushing through your meal to get to the next moment. Make it a point to pay attention, not just to the flavor of your food but to the whole experience. Eating a meal is supposed to be pleasurable. Take it all in.

Isn't Fasting Bad for Women?

There is a commonly held belief that fasting is bad for women, and while this can be true for some women, it's not a blanket statement that can be applied to all women. This theory developed due to the fact that intermittent fasting has the potential to cause a hormonal imbalance in some women if the fasting is not done properly; but when the proper care and precautions are taken, women can fast successfully.

Because women's bodies were physiologically designed to carry babies, they're more sensitive to potential starvation than men. If a woman's body senses any impending starvation, it will respond by increasing the hormones leptin and ghrelin, which work together to control hunger. This hormonal response is the female body's way of protecting a developing fetus, even if a woman is not currently pregnant.

Although it's possible to ignore the hunger signals from ghrelin and leptin, it becomes increasingly difficult, especially as the body revolts and starts to produce more of these hormones. If a woman gives in to the hunger in an unhealthy way—by overeating or consuming unhealthy foods—this can cause a cascade of other hormonal issues involving insulin.

This process can also shut down the reproductive system. If your body thinks it doesn't have enough food to survive, it might shut down the ability to conceive to protect a potential pregnancy. This is why fasting is not recommended during pregnancy or for women who are trying to become pregnant.

There is something called the hypothalamic-pituitary-gonadal (HPG) axis, which controls the endocrine glands involved in ovulation. The first part of the ovulation process is the release of gonadotropin releasing hormone (GnRH) from the hypothalamus. The release of GnRH then triggers the pituitary gland to release both follicular stimulating hormone (FSH) and luteinizing hormone (LH). In women, the release of FSH and LH trigger the ovaries and the production of estrogen and progesterone. The increase in estrogen and progesterone is what causes the release of a mature egg (ovulation). This hormonal cascade is very precise and specific, and in healthy women it happens in a regular cycle. However, GnRH is extremely sensitive to environmental and outside factors and can be thrown off by fasting.

Men have an HPG axis, too, but the process works a little differently. Instead of acting on the ovaries (which men don't have), FSH and LH act on the testes and trigger the production of testosterone and sperm. The HPG axis in men is not as sensitive to fasting, however, because men's bodies aren't designed to carry children. Thus, the body's protection alert is not triggered as easily.

Crescendo Fasting

This doesn't mean that intermittent fasting isn't right for you if you're a woman; it just means that you should ease into it a little more carefully. If you're a woman who's fasting for the first time, trying to figure out if it's right for you, you may want to start with crescendo fasting.

With crescendo fasting, you only fast for twelve to sixteen hours a few days per week, rather than every day. These fast days should be nonconsecutive (Tuesday, Thursday, and Saturday, for example). On fasting days, you should engage only in light exercise, like yoga or walking. Strenuous exercise, like strength training, should be reserved for nonfasting days, when you're eating normally. It's also important to drink plenty of water—the typical recommendation is the equivalent of half of your body weight in ounces, so if you weigh 140 pounds, you should drink a minimum of 70 ounces of water each day. Of course, the amount of water you need depends on a variety of factors, including your age, weight, activity level, and the amount of coffee you drink, but you should use this equation as a baseline.

If you feel good after crescendo fasting for a couple of weeks, you can add in another day of fasting and see how your body reacts. If you still feel good, you can add in more days until you reach your fasting goals. The main point of crescendo fasting is to ease in slowly and avoid shocking the body too much at once.

CHAPTER 7

Breakfast

Breakfast Casserole

You can prepare this delicious casserole a day or two in advance so you have a quick breakfast ready to go that doesn't require any extra prep.

INGREDIENTS | SERVES 4

1 pound 85 percent lean ground beef
1 small yellow onion, peeled and diced
1 teaspoon freshly ground black pepper
1 teaspoon garlic powder
1 teaspoon red pepper flakes
12 large eggs
1 cup unsweetened full-fat coconut milk
1 tablespoon coconut oil
1 small butternut squash, peeled, seeded, and sliced

1. In a large skillet over medium heat, start cooking ground beef. Add onion and spices, cooking 10 minutes until onions are soft.
2. In a large bowl, whip together eggs and milk.
3. Grease the inside of a 4–6-quart slow cooker with coconut oil. Add in squash, beef and onion mixture, and egg and milk mixture. Stir and make sure that beef and onion mixture is completely covered by egg and milk mixture. Cook on low heat 10 hours.
4. Scoop out, slice, and serve warm.

Per Serving: | Calories: 581 | Fat: 37.4g | Protein: 41.3g | Sodium: 288mg | Fiber: 1.6g | Carbohydrates: 11.4g | Net Carbohydrates: 9.8g | Sugar: 2.5g

Autumn Breakfast Chia Bowl

This Autumn Breakfast Chia Bowl contains cranberry and cinnamon flavors reminiscent of the fall, but it can be enjoyed any time of the year.

* Under 500 Calories *

INGREDIENTS | SERVES 2

3 cups cold water
¼ teaspoon salt
1 cup gluten-free steel-cut oats
½ cup unsweetened almond milk
3 tablespoons chia seeds
1 tablespoon halved macadamia nuts
1 tablespoon raw sliced almonds
½ teaspoon ground cinnamon
1 tablespoon no-sugar-added dried cranberries

1. In a medium saucepan, bring water and salt to a boil on high heat, then add oats. Reduce heat to medium-low, add milk, and stir.
2. Add chia seeds, macadamia nuts, almonds, cinnamon, and cranberries to pan and stir.
3. Cover and cook on medium-low heat 20 minutes, stirring occasionally until chia seeds become soft and gel-like. Serve immediately.

Per Serving: | Calories: 471 | Fat: 15.6g | Protein: 17.8g | Sodium: 352mg | Fiber: 16.8g | Carbohydrates: 67.2g | Net Carbohydrates: 50.4g | Sugar: 0.6g

Turkey, Egg White, and Hash Brown Bake

You can beat any craving for a hearty, but still healthy, breakfast with this satisfying dish. Quick and easy to whip up, this bake is perfect for your first meal—or any meal—of the day.

* Under 500 Calories *

INGREDIENTS | SERVES 16

Olive oil cooking spray
1 tablespoon olive oil
1 pound 85 percent lean ground turkey
1 pound Russet potatoes, peeled and shredded
12 large eggs
1½ teaspoons salt
1½ teaspoons freshly ground black pepper
½ teaspoon ground cayenne pepper

1. Preheat oven to 375°F.
2. Grease a 9" × 13" glass casserole dish with cooking spray.
3. Heat oil in a skillet over medium heat 1 minute. Add ground turkey and cook until no longer pink, about 6 minutes.
4. Transfer cooked turkey to a large bowl and combine with remaining ingredients. Mix well.
5. Pour mixture into prepared baking dish. Bake 40 minutes until top is set and an inserted toothpick comes out clean.
6. Allow to cool 5 minutes, then cut into 16 pieces and serve.

Per Serving: | Calories: 137 | Fat: 7.4g | Protein: 10.7g | Sodium: 344mg | Fiber: 0.5g | Carbohydrates: 5.1g | Net Carbohydrates: 4.6g | Sugar: 0.4g

Cran-Orange Oatmeal

If your standard oatmeal recipe feels a bit bland, try this revamped version! Tart cranberries and fresh orange add extra vitamins and minerals—and a zesty flavor that kicks things up a notch.

* Under 500 Calories *

INGREDIENTS | SERVES 2

1 cup freshly squeezed orange juice
½ cup water
1 cup fresh cranberries
2 cups gluten-free rolled oats
1 tablespoon maple syrup
1 tablespoon freshly grated orange zest

1. Combine orange juice, water, and cranberries in a medium saucepan over medium heat. Bring to a simmer, about 5 minutes.
2. Add oats and simmer, stirring constantly, until thickened, about 8 minutes. Remove from heat and stir in maple syrup.
3. Divide oatmeal into two bowls, garnish with orange zest, and serve immediately.

Per Serving: | Calories: 487 | Fat: 7.2g | Protein: 15.1g | Sodium: 3mg | Fiber: 12.9g | Carbohydrates: 90.5g | Net Carbohydrates: 77.6g | Sugar: 20.5g

South of the Border Scrambler

Short on time? This scrambled version of huevos rancheros can be made in minutes. If you want a kick, spice it up with some sliced jalapeños.

* Under 500 Calories *

INGREDIENTS | SERVES 2

4 large eggs
½ teaspoon salt
¼ teaspoon freshly ground black pepper
1 teaspoon olive oil
¼ cup no-sugar-added salsa
½ large avocado, diced
¼ cup chopped fresh cilantro

1. Whisk eggs, salt, and pepper together in a medium bowl.
2. Heat olive oil 30 seconds in a medium skillet over medium heat. Add eggs and scramble until cooked, about 4 minutes.
3. Transfer to two bowls and top each with ⅛ cup salsa, ¼ diced avocado, and ⅛ cup cilantro. Serve immediately.

Per Serving: | Calories: 239 | Fat: 15.6g | Protein: 13.3g | Sodium: 956mg | Fiber: 2.8g | Carbohydrates: 6.9g | Net Carbohydrates: 4.1g | Sugar: 2.5g

Simple Salsa Recipe

Here's a simple recipe for homemade salsa: combine 2 tomatoes, ½ seeded jalapeño, 2 cilantro branches, the juice of ½ lemon, ¼ teaspoon salt, and ⅛ teaspoon pepper. Put all ingredients in a food processor and pulse until combined.

Tomato Spinach Frittata Muffins

Easy to make and fun to bake! Enjoy frittata in a new way with these muffins.

* Under 500 Calories *

INGREDIENTS | SERVES 12

2 cups finely chopped fresh spinach
1½ cups halved cherry tomatoes
1 scallion, trimmed and finely chopped, green part only
10 large eggs
2 tablespoons unsweetened full-fat coconut milk
1 teaspoon dried ground oregano
⅛ teaspoon salt
¼ teaspoon freshly ground black pepper

1. Preheat oven to 375°F. Grease a 12-cup muffin pan with cooking spray.
2. Divide spinach, tomatoes, and scallion evenly and place in muffin cups.
3. In a medium bowl, whisk together eggs, milk, oregano, salt, and pepper. Pour egg mixture evenly into each muffin cup.
4. Bake 20 minutes until eggs are completely set. Serve.

Per Serving: | Calories: 69 | Fat: 4.2g | Protein: 5.6g | Sodium: 88mg | Fiber: 0.4g | Carbohydrates: 1.4g | Net Carbohydrates: 1.0g | Sugar: 0.7g

You Can Eat the Green!

Whole onions, shallots, and the white part of spring onions (scallions) are high in FODMAPs because they contain the "O" in FODMAPs: oligosaccharides (fructans). Fructans are made of fructose molecule chains that the body has trouble absorbing. The green parts of the scallion, however, are low in FODMAPs, so you'll want to choose the green if you are sensitive to FODMAPs.

Flourless Banana Cinnamon Pancakes

These are the easiest and healthiest pancakes you will ever make. They're gluten-free and contain ingredients that you probably have on hand already.

* Under 500 Calories *

INGREDIENTS | SERVES 1

1 large egg
½ ripe medium banana, mashed well
1 teaspoon chia seeds
1 teaspoon ground cinnamon
1 tablespoon coconut oil

1. In a large glass measuring cup or blender on low speed, mix together egg, banana, chia seeds, and cinnamon until smooth.
2. Heat oil in a medium skillet over medium heat. Pour two small circles of batter onto skillet and cook until bubbly on top and golden on bottom, about 4 minutes. Flip and cook an additional 2 minutes. Repeat with remaining batter.

Per Serving: | Calories: 262 | Fat: 18.3g | Protein: 7.6g | Sodium: 71mg | Fiber: 4.1g | Carbohydrates: 17.4g | Net Carbohydrates: 13.3g | Sugar: 7.5g

Looking for More Fun Flavor Combinations?

Try adding alcohol-free vanilla or almond extract, shredded unsweetened coconut, walnuts, slivered almonds, ground macadamia nuts, pumpkin seeds, pumpkin purée, or no-sugar-added dried cranberries to the batter.

Coconut Cacao Hazelnut Smoothie Bowl

This nutty and chocolaty bowl is delicious and loaded with healthy fats and micronutrients. Enjoy it as your first meal of the day to get a jump-start on your daily nutrient needs.

* Under 500 Calories *

INGREDIENTS | SERVES 1

1 tablespoon shredded unsweetened coconut
1 cup unsweetened almond milk
1 frozen ripe medium banana
2 teaspoons raw unsweetened cacao powder
1½ teaspoons pure maple syrup
⅛ teaspoon sea salt
6 ice cubes (approximately ½ cup)
5 hazelnuts, shelled and chopped
1 tablespoon shelled pumpkin seeds

1. Toast coconut in a small skillet over medium heat, stirring frequently until flakes are golden brown, about 3 minutes. Set aside.
2. Add milk, banana, cacao, maple syrup, and salt to blender with ice and blend until smooth. Add more ice if desired to make mixture thicker.
3. Pour mixture into a serving bowl and top with hazelnuts, pumpkin seeds, and toasted coconut. Serve.

Per Serving: | Calories: 294 | Fat: 14.2g | Protein: 6.5g | Sodium: 379mg | Fiber: 6.6g | Carbohydrates: 41.1g | Net Carbohydrates: 34.5g | Sugar: 21.3g

Cacao versus Cocoa

Cacao and cocoa come from the same plant, but the major difference is in how they're processed. Cacao is minimally processed and made by cold-pressing cacao beans. Cocoa starts out as cacao, but is heated at much higher temperatures than cacao, which results in a sweeter flavor. Both cacao and cocoa have health benefits, but the heat used during the processing of cocoa destroys some of the antioxidants and enzymes in it, making cacao a nutritionally superior choice.

Overnight Almond Butter Pumpkin Spice Oats

You will love digging into these hearty and delicious pumpkin oats! This dish is perfect for tiding you over during a busy day.

* Under 500 Calories *

INGREDIENTS | SERVES 2

½ cup gluten-free rolled oats
¼ cup unsweetened almond milk
¼ cup pumpkin purée
½ teaspoon pumpkin pie spice
½ teaspoon alcohol-free vanilla extract
½ teaspoon ground cinnamon
1 tablespoon pure maple syrup
2 tablespoons unsalted, no-sugar-added almond butter
2 tablespoons chopped walnuts

1. In a medium bowl, combine oats and milk and stir. Add pumpkin purée, pumpkin pie spice, vanilla, cinnamon, and maple syrup. Stir.
2. Spoon half of oats mixture into each of two small canning jars. Add 1 tablespoon almond butter on top of oats in each jar. Divide remaining oats on top of almond butter. Cover with jar lids. Refrigerate overnight.
3. In the morning, top with walnuts and enjoy! Mixture can be refrigerated up to 3 days.

Per Serving: | Calories: 288 | Fat: 14.9g | Protein: 8.4g | Sodium: 25mg | Fiber: 5.9g | Carbohydrates: 30.4g | Net Carbohydrates: 24.5g | Sugar: 8.9g

Overnight Oats Have So Many Possibilities!

Overnight oats are so easy to make, and there are several different variations you can try with any of your favorite ingredients. Start with a base of oats and your favorite non-dairy milk, and then add any combination of nuts, berries, spices, and a dash of a healthy sweetener (like pure maple syrup or honey). Overnight oats keep well in the refrigerator, so you can make a few at a time and keep them in jars, ready to grab on your way out the door.

Mini Quiche

These promise a tasty protein-packed breakfast—or any meal of the day—and can be made in bulk to last for the week.

* Under 500 Calories *

INGREDIENTS | SERVES 8

6 large eggs
6 slices nitrate- and nitrite-free bacon
1 tablespoon pure olive oil
½ cup chopped fresh broccoli florets
½ cup sliced white mushrooms
½ cup peeled and diced yellow onions
½ cup seeded and diced red bell peppers

1. Preheat oven to 325°F. Line muffin tin with 8 foil cups.
2. Whisk together eggs and set aside.
3. Cook bacon until crisp, about 5 minutes, then let cool 5 minutes on a paper towel before chopping into ½" pieces.
4. Add oil to medium sauté pan over medium-high heat. Sauté remaining ingredients 5 minutes.
5. Pour eggs into foil cups, filling each cup ⅔ of the way.
6. Divide bacon and vegetables evenly into each cup.
7. Bake 25 minutes until golden brown. Serve.

Per Serving: | Calories: 162 | Fat: 12.7g | Protein: 7.8g | Sodium: 194mg | Fiber: 0.4g | Carbohydrate: 1.8g | Net Carbohydrates: 1.4g | Sugar: 1.1g

Spicy Kale Scramble

This great post-workout breakfast provides healthy proteins and greens—with a kick!

* Under 500 Calories *

INGREDIENTS | SERVES 1

1 tablespoon olive oil
1 cup chopped fresh kale
3 large eggs, whisked
2 teaspoons ground turmeric
½ teaspoon salt
¼ teaspoon freshly ground black pepper
⅛ teaspoon ground cayenne pepper

1. Heat olive oil in a medium skillet over medium heat 1 minute. Add kale and cook until wilted, about 3 minutes.
2. Add whisked eggs to skillet, along with remaining ingredients. Scramble eggs until cooked through, about 4 minutes.
3. Serve immediately.

Per Serving: | Calories: 359 | Fat: 26.5g | Protein: 20.2g | Sodium: 1,382mg | Fiber: 2.1g | Carbohydrates: 7.0g | Net Carbohydrates: 4.9g | Sugar: 1.1g

Add More Greens

This is a basic recipe that you can make even more nutritious by adding your favorite greens. Spinach, arugula, and collard greens are all great choices.

Vegetarian Hash

This version of an old favorite is bursting with flavor. It can be eaten as a side dish or as an entrée.

*** Under 500 Calories ***

INGREDIENTS | SERVES 6

1½ pounds Russet potatoes, peeled and large-diced

1 medium poblano (or other mild chili pepper), halved and seeded

2 medium red bell peppers, stemmed, halved, and seeded

1 medium red onion, peeled and thickly sliced

½ teaspoon olive oil

1 tablespoon chili powder

¼ teaspoon freshly cracked black peppercorns

¼ bunch fresh cilantro, chopped

¼ teaspoon salt

1. Preheat oven to 400°F.
2. Toss potatoes, peppers, and onions in oil, then drain on a rack. Place vegetables on an ungreased baking sheet and season with chili powder and black pepper; roast until fork-tender. (Times will vary; check with fork at 5-minute intervals.)
3. Large-dice peppers and onions. Combine potatoes, peppers, onions, and cilantro. Season with salt and serve.

Per Serving: | Calories: 119 | Fat: 0.9g | Protein: 2.9g | Sodium: 143mg | Fiber: 3.7g | Carbohydrates: 26.2g | Net Carbohydrates: 22.5g | Sugar: 4.1g

Roughly Cracked Black Pepper

Like many seeds, black pepper's true flavor remains locked inside until it's smashed. Place about ten peppercorns at a time on a flat, hard surface. Using a small saucepot or small skillet, apply pressure with the heel of your hand to break the seeds a few at a time. Use it as you would ground black pepper.

Chicken Sausage Patties

These delicious sausages pair well with a side of poached eggs and Vegetarian Hash. Serve with spicy chutney for an added kick.

* Under 500 Calories *

INGREDIENTS | YIELDS 24 PATTIES

3 pounds ground chicken

1 medium yellow onion, peeled and finely minced

½ cup finely chopped fresh flat-leaf parsley

1 tablespoon chopped fresh sage (or 2 teaspoons dry ground sage)

6 cloves garlic, peeled and minced

1 tablespoon peeled and minced fresh ginger (or 2 teaspoons dry ground ginger)

2 teaspoons red pepper flakes

1 teaspoon ground cloves

1 teaspoon ground white pepper

4 tablespoons olive oil

1. In a large mixing bowl, combine all ingredients; mix well by hand.
2. Form mixture into 24 patties that are approximately 2" round.
3. Heat the oil in a large sauté pan until hot, about 30 seconds. Sauté patties over medium heat approximately 5 minutes on each side, until cooked through.

Per Serving: 1 patty | Calories: 105 | Fat: 6.4g | Protein: 10.1g | Sodium: 35mg | Fiber: 0.2g | Carbohydrates: 1.0g | Net Carbohydrates: 0.8g | Sugar: 0.2g

Artichoke and Cheese Squares

These rich vegetable cakes are easy to prepare and can be made up to three days ahead of time.

*** Under 500 Calories ***

INGREDIENTS | SERVES 8

1 (12-ounce) jar marinated artichoke hearts, drained and chopped, liquid reserved
1 small yellow onion, peeled and finely chopped
2 cloves garlic, peeled and finely minced
4 large eggs, beaten
2 tablespoons coconut flour
½ teaspoon salt
¼ teaspoon freshly ground black pepper
¼ teaspoon dried ground oregano
¼ teaspoon Tabasco
8 ounces shredded Monterey jack cheese
2 tablespoons chopped fresh flat-leaf parsley

1. Preheat oven to 325°F.
2. Heat artichoke liquid in a medium skillet over medium heat 1 minute. Sauté onion and garlic in skillet 5 minutes until onions are translucent.
3. In a mixing bowl, combine eggs, flour, salt, pepper, oregano, and Tabasco. Mix in cheese, parsley, artichokes, onion, and garlic.
4. Pour mixture into a 7" × 11" baking dish. Bake 30 minutes until egg is set. Cool 10 minutes. Cut into squares and serve at room temperature, or reheat at 325°F 10 minutes and serve warm.

Per Serving: | Calories: 175 | Fat: 11.2g | Protein: 12.1g | Sodium: 665mg | Fiber: 2.3g | Carbohydrates: 5.5g | Net Carbohydrates: 3.2g | Sugar: 1.0g

Roasted Vegetable Frittata

This Roasted Vegetable Frittata can be made ahead and served at slightly above room temperature. It's the perfect way to utilize any leftover vegetables, so feel free to get creative with whatever is in your refrigerator.

* Under 500 Calories *

INGREDIENTS | SERVES 8

1 medium zucchini, quartered lengthwise and cut into chunks
1 medium yellow squash, quartered lengthwise
1 cup small white mushrooms, roughly chopped
1 small Italian eggplant (or ¼ a regular eggplant), cut into large chunks
2 tablespoons olive oil
9 large eggs, beaten
¾ cup unsweetened almond milk
½ teaspoon salt
2 tablespoons unsalted grass-fed butter
1 medium Russet potato, peeled, baked and diced
1 medium yellow onion, peeled and chopped
1 tablespoon chopped fresh flat-leaf parsley
½ cup diced tomato (about 1 large)
1 cup shredded cheese (Monterey jack, Cheddar, or Havarti)
¼ teaspoon freshly ground black pepper

1. Preheat oven to 400°F. Toss together zucchini, yellow squash, mushrooms, and eggplant with olive oil.
2. Spread mixture on an ungreased baking sheet or in roasting pan. Roast in oven until tender, about 20 minutes. Remove vegetable mixture and raise oven temperature to 450°F.
3. In a medium bowl, whisk together eggs, milk, and salt. In an oven-safe, 12" nonstick skillet, melt butter over medium heat, about 20 seconds.
4. Add potatoes, onions, and parsley to skillet; cook until onions are softened and potatoes are slightly browned, about 10 minutes.
5. Add roasted vegetables and egg mixture to skillet. Cook, stirring with a wooden spoon, approximately 4 minutes until mixture begins to thicken but is still mostly liquid.
6. Stir in tomatoes and cheese. Season with pepper. Place pan on center rack of oven and bake until frittata puffs slightly and begins to brown on top, about 15 minutes.
7. Remove skillet from oven and transfer frittata to a serving plate. Allow it to rest 5 minutes before cutting into 8 wedges and serving.

Per Serving: | Calories: 233 | Fat: 15.7g | Protein: 12.3g | Sodium: 340mg | Fiber: 1.9g | Carbohydrates: 9.6g | Net Carbohydrates: 7.7g | Sugar: 3.5g

Tomato and Leek Frittata

Leeks add a mild taste to this frittata, but you can also use onions in their place. Serve this frittata garnished with extra goat cheese, tomato slices, and sliced scallions for an added flair.

* Under 500 Calories *

INGREDIENTS | SERVES 2

3 teaspoons olive oil, divided
½ cup chopped leek greens
½ teaspoon sea salt, divided
½ teaspoon freshly ground black pepper, divided
½ cup whole grape tomatoes
¼ cup capers, drained and rinsed
3 egg whites
1 teaspoon dried herbes de Provence
1 teaspoon dried thyme
2 egg yolks
2 ounces goat cheese, crumbled

1. Preheat oven to 350°F.
2. Heat 2 teaspoons oil in a 10" oven-safe, nonstick skillet over medium heat 1 minute. Add leeks, ¼ teaspoon salt, and ¼ teaspoon pepper to skillet. Cook 5 minutes.
3. Stir in grape tomatoes and capers. Cover and cook 3 minutes. Transfer mixture to a small bowl.
4. In a medium bowl, quickly beat egg whites with herbes de Provence, thyme, and remaining salt and pepper. Whisk in egg yolks until mixture is fluffy.
5. Brush skillet with remaining oil. Add seasoned eggs, cooked tomato mixture, and goat cheese. Cook over medium heat 4 minutes.
6. Transfer skillet to oven; bake 20 minutes until eggs are set. To check, cut a small slit in center of frittata. Slice and serve.

Per Serving: | Calories: 258 | Fat: 18.0g | Protein: 15.4g | Sodium: 991mg | Fiber: 1.7g | Carbohydrates: 7.1g | Net Carbohydrates: 5.4g | Sugar: 2.4g

Raspberry Banana Mint Chia Pudding

Raspberry and mint go perfectly together and make this pudding great for breakfast—or any time of the day!

*** Under 500 Calories ***

INGREDIENTS | SERVES 2

½ cup canned unsweetened full-fat coconut milk

½ cup unsweetened almond milk

¼ cup chia seeds

1 teaspoon alcohol-free mint extract

1 tablespoon pure maple syrup

½ ripe medium banana, sliced

10 fresh raspberries

2 tablespoons shredded unsweetened coconut

2 whole fresh mint leaves

1. Add milks, chia seeds, mint extract, and maple syrup to a jar and mix well. Cover and refrigerate, mixing every 2 hours throughout the day, then refrigerate overnight.
2. Add banana slices to jar, followed by raspberries, coconut, and mint leaves. Enjoy immediately or refrigerate up to 2 days.

Per Serving: | Calories: 313 | Fat: 21.2g | Protein: 5.5g | Sodium: 56mg | Fiber: 9.7g | Carbohydrates: 26.9g | Net Carbohydrates: 17.2g | Sugar: 10.8g

Gut-Friendly Smoothie

Although fasting helps reduce inflammation on its own, adding turmeric to your diet can boost the effect even more. Curcumin, the main compound in turmeric, has been shown to have a significant anti-inflammatory effect.

INGREDIENTS | SERVES 1

1 cup canned unsweetened full-fat coconut milk
1 tablespoon coconut oil
1 tablespoon chia seeds
½ ripe medium banana
½ teaspoon ground turmeric
½ teaspoon ground cinnamon

Blend all ingredients thoroughly in a blender and enjoy immediately.

Per Serving: | Calories: 676 | Fat: 61.6g | Protein: 7.3g | Sodium: 30mg | Fiber: 6.5g | Carbohydrates: 26.7g | Net Carbohydrates: 20.2g | Sugar: 7.3g

Pineapple Turmeric Smoothie

This yummy, anti-inflammatory smoothie is refreshing, smooth, and easy on the stomach, so it's a great way to break your fast in the morning.

* Under 500 Calories *

INGREDIENTS | SERVES 1

1 cup coconut water
6 ice cubes (approximately ½ cup)
1 cup chopped fresh pineapple
½ teaspoon ground turmeric
½ teaspoon ground cinnamon
¼ teaspoon freshly ground black pepper
1 tablespoon chia seeds
1 tablespoon shredded unsweetened coconut
¼ teaspoon freshly grated ginger
Juice of ½ medium lime

Place coconut water and ice in a blender. Add remaining ingredients and blend until smooth. Add more ice if desired. Serve immediately.

Per Serving: | Calories: 226 | Fat: 7.0g | Protein: 5.1g | Sodium: 254mg | Fiber: 11.1g | Carbohydrates: 40.5g | Net Carbohydrates: 29.4g | Sugar: 22.9g

Breakfast Salad

Salad isn't just for lunch and dinner anymore. You can enjoy this filling dish around the clock!

INGREDIENTS | SERVES 1

3 cups fresh baby spinach

4 large eggs, hard-boiled, peeled, and quartered

2 slices nitrate- and nitrite-free bacon, cooked and chopped

½ cup sliced cucumber

½ medium avocado, peeled, pitted, and diced

½ medium apple, cored and sliced

Juice of ½ medium lemon

1. Arrange spinach leaves on a plate and top with eggs and bacon. Add cucumber, avocado, and apple slices to salad.
2. Squeeze fresh lemon juice over salad. Serve immediately.

Per Serving: | Calories: 598 | Fat: 34.8g | Protein: 37.5g | Sodium: 712mg | Fiber: 8.0g | Carbohydrate: 25.0g | Net Carbohydrates: 17.0g | Sugar: 12.2g

Bacon and Vegetable Omelet

Bacon and eggs are a breakfast tradition. This omelet combines the two breakfast favorites with vegetables to help you optimize your micronutrient intake during your feeding times.

INGREDIENTS | SERVES 2

6 slices nitrate- and nitrite-free bacon, diced

1 medium yellow summer squash, chopped

1 cup white mushrooms, sliced

1 medium zucchini, chopped

¼ cup fresh basil leaves, chopped

2 tablespoons olive oil

8 large eggs, beaten

1. In a large sauté pan, cook bacon until crispy, about 5 minutes. Add vegetables and basil to the pan and sauté until tender, approximately 8 minutes.
2. Heat olive oil in a second sauté pan over medium heat, about 1 minute.
3. Add eggs to second pan and cook 3 minutes on each side.
4. Place vegetable and bacon mixture on one-half of eggs and fold over other half to enclose filling. Serve.

Per Serving: | Calories: 606 | Fat: 42.5g | Protein: 40.4g | Sodium: 875mg | Fiber: 2.5g | Carbohydrate: 9.6g | Net Carbohydrates: 7.1g | Sugar: 6.1g

Strawberry Banana Pancakes

This pancake is a fun way to get some variety in your breakfast. It's not only delicious, it's also quick and easy to make!

* Under 500 Calories *

INGREDIENTS | SERVES 1

Avocado oil cooking spray
3 egg whites, lightly beaten
1 tablespoon almond butter
1 ripe medium banana, sliced
4 fresh strawberries, hulled and sliced
½ teaspoon ground cinnamon

1. Heat a small frying pan coated with avocado oil cooking spray on medium-low heat 1 minute.
2. In a medium bowl, mix well together egg whites and almond butter, then add banana and strawberries.
3. Pour mixture into pan, cover with lid, and cook 3 minutes.
4. Flip pancake to brown on other side 2 minutes.
5. Serve warm and garnish with cinnamon sprinkled on top.

Per Serving: | Calories: 272 | Fat: 8.4g | Protein: 15.8g | Sodium: 166mg | Fiber: 6.4g | Carbohydrate: 35.4g | Net Carbohydrates: 28.1g | Sugar: 18.2g

Salmon Omelet

This savory omelet is full of omega-3 fatty acids. It will surely become a breakfast staple.

* Under 500 Calories *

INGREDIENTS | SERVES 2

2 tablespoons olive oil
¼ cup trimmed and chopped scallions
1 cup trimmed and chopped asparagus
1 tablespoon chopped fresh dill
6 ounces canned salmon
6 large eggs, beaten

1. In a large skillet, combine olive oil, scallions, asparagus, and dill. Sauté over medium-high heat until asparagus is soft, about 10 minutes, then remove mixture from skillet and set aside.
2. In same skillet sauté salmon until flaky, about 10 minutes, depending on thickness of salmon. Remove from skillet and set aside.
3. Wipe out skillet with a paper towel and cook eggs on both sides until lightly browned, about 5 minutes each side.
4. Place salmon and asparagus mixture on one-half of eggs, fold other half over to enclose filling. Serve.

Per Serving: | Calories: 484 | Fat: 30.2g | Protein: 42.9g | Sodium: 544mg | Fiber: 1.7g | Carbohydrate: 4.6g | Net Carbohydrates: 2.9g | Sugar: 2.1g

Old-Fashioned Sweet Potato Hash Browns

These sweet potato hash browns are not only a perfect breakfast component, they're also delicious as a side for any meal. If you make extra, you'll have them ready to go when it's time to break your fast but you don't feel like cooking.

* Under 500 Calories *

INGREDIENTS | SERVES 6

3 tablespoons coconut oil

3 medium sweet potatoes, peeled and grated

1 tablespoon ground cinnamon

1. Heat coconut oil in a large sauté pan over medium-high heat 1 minute.
2. Cook sweet potatoes in oil 7 minutes, stirring often.
3. Transfer potatoes to serving dish, sprinkle with cinnamon, and serve.

Per Serving: | Calories: 114 | Fat: 5.9g | Protein: 1.1g | Sodium: 20mg | Fiber: 2.6g | Carbohydrate: 14.4g | Net Carbohydrates: 11.8g | Sugar: 4.4g

Garlicky Vegetable-Packed Omelet

Delicious vegetables and garlic combine with fluffy eggs and egg whites to make a simple, satisfying, and savory meal that will start any day off right! Protein-packed and rich in complex carbohydrates from the vegetables, this is a tasty way to get some valuable nutrition.

* Under 500 Calories *

INGREDIENTS | SERVES 1

Olive oil cooking spray
¼ cup peeled and chopped yellow onion
¼ cup sliced white mushrooms
2 tablespoons filtered water
2 teaspoons garlic powder
¼ cup torn fresh spinach leaves
3 large eggs

1. Coat a small frying pan with olive oil cooking spray and heat over medium heat 1 minute.
2. Add onions and sauté 1 minute. Add mushrooms and water and continue sautéing until mushrooms are softened, about 4 minutes.
3. Sprinkle garlic powder on onion-mushroom mixture and stir in spinach leaves.
4. Whisk together eggs and pour egg mixture over sautéed vegetables.
5. Immediately begin pulling outer edges of mixture into the center for one turn around the whole pan. Let omelet cook untouched 2 minutes.
6. Slide a spatula under omelet, gently lifting the center from the pan. Once omelet is balancing on spatula, quickly flip omelet over onto other side.
7. Continue cooking omelet another 5 minutes until no juices remain when omelet is pressed on. Fold eggs over. Remove from heat and enjoy.

Per Serving: | Calories: 254 | Fat: 13.1g | Protein: 21.1g | Sodium: 222mg | Fiber: 1.6g | Carbohydrates: 10.2g | Net Carbohydrates: 8.6g | Sugar: 2.8g

Gracious Garlic

A member of the lily flower family, garlic is a beautiful plant that can give your meal a tantalizing aroma and a unique flavor. Use just a single clove from the bulb of this versatile plant to dress up boring dishes or add a savory new flavor.

Very Vegetable Frittata

Packed with loads of protein from the egg whites and yolks and rich in carbohydrates from all of the fresh vegetables, this great-tasting frittata will leave you full and energized. Customize it using your favorite vegetables!

* Under 500 Calories *

INGREDIENTS | SERVES 4

Olive oil cooking spray
½ cup chopped fresh broccoli florets
½ cup diced white mushrooms
½ cup seeded and chopped yellow bell pepper
¼ yellow onion, peeled and finely chopped
¼ cup filtered water
8 large eggs
1 tablespoon garlic powder
1 teaspoon sea salt
2 teaspoons freshly ground black pepper

1. Preheat oven to 350°F. Grease a large oven-safe skillet with olive oil cooking spray and preheat over medium heat 1 minute.
2. Combine broccoli, mushrooms, bell pepper, and onions in skillet with water and cook until tender but not soft, about 5 minutes.
3. Whisk together eggs, garlic powder, salt, and black pepper and pour over vegetable mixture.
4. Cook until center of mixture begins to shake and bubble from heat, about 4 minutes.
5. Remove skillet from heat and place in preheated oven 15 minutes, until center of mixture is set and an inserted fork comes out clean. Cut into wedges and serve.

Per Serving: | Calories: 166 | Fat: 8.8g | Protein: 13.9g | Sodium: 536mg | Fiber: 1.1g | Carbohydrates: 5.7g | Net Carbohydrates: 4.6g | Sugar: 1.7g

Heavenly Hash Browns

The classic version of this breakfast staple gets a complete overhaul in this delicious hash browns recipe. By using clean, fresh ingredients and replacing the not-so-healthy oils with a small amount of olive oil, you can enjoy every last bite of these hearty hash browns.

* Under 500 Calories *

INGREDIENTS | SERVES 6

Olive oil cooking spray
3 medium Idaho potatoes, scrubbed and shredded
1 small yellow onion, peeled and minced
1 large egg
1 teaspoon garlic powder
¼ teaspoon sea salt
¼ teaspoon freshly ground black pepper
1 tablespoon olive oil

1. Grease a large skillet with olive oil cooking spray and preheat over medium heat 1 minute.
2. In a large mixing bowl, combine shredded potatoes, onions, egg, and garlic powder and mix until thoroughly blended. Add salt and pepper.
3. Form potato mixture into dense patties, using ½ cup of mixture for each patty.
4. Heat olive oil in skillet 1 minute and add two hash brown patties. Cook 5 minutes until golden brown.
5. Flip patties and continue cooking another 4 minutes until golden brown on both sides and completely cooked through. Remove and repeat process with remaining patties.

Per Serving: | Calories: 120 | Fat: 3.0g | Protein: 3.4g | Sodium: 83mg | Fiber: 2.6g | Carbohydrates: 20.2g | Net Carbohydrates: 17.6g | Sugar: 1.4g

Pumpkin Spice Smoothie

If you're looking for an escape from the usual fruit smoothie, mix things up with this delicious pumpkin pie in a glass! Raw ingredients and aromatic spices make this clean smoothie one of the most delicious and healthy breakfast options around.

* Under 500 Calories *

INGREDIENTS | SERVES 2

1 cup canned sweet potato purée
1 cup unsweetened vanilla almond milk
1 teaspoon ground cloves
1 teaspoon ground ginger
1 teaspoon ground cinnamon
24 ice cubes (approximately 2 cups)

1. Combine sweet potato purée, milk, and spices in a blender with half of ice and blend until thoroughly combined.
2. Add remaining ice gradually and blend until desired consistency.

Per Serving: | Calories: 150 | Fat: 1.8g | Protein: 3.2g | Sodium: 188mg | Fiber: 3.7g | Carbohydrates: 32.6g | Net Carbohydrates: 28.9g | Sugar: 7.2g

Huevos Rancheros Without Tortillas

This is a classic dish from south of the border. If you eat grains, you can use brown rice tortillas to turn these into breakfast burritos.

* Under 500 Calories *

INGREDIENTS | SERVES 2

3 tablespoons olive oil, divided
2 medium vine-ripened tomatoes, finely chopped
2 small shallots, finely chopped
½ teaspoon sea salt, divided
2 large eggs
¼ teaspoon freshly ground pepper
¼ cup fresh cilantro leaves
1 medium jalapeño pepper, stemmed, seeded, and finely chopped

1. Heat 2 tablespoons oil in a nonstick pan over medium heat 1 minute.
2. Add tomatoes and shallots to pan and season with ¼ teaspoon salt. Cover pan and let cook, stirring occasionally about 5 minutes until shallots are limp. Set mixture aside.
3. Heat remaining tablespoon of oil in medium nonstick skillet over medium heat 1 minute.
4. Crack eggs into skillet and cook sunny-side up until whites are set and yolks are still soft, about 2 minutes. If you prefer yolks fully cooked, cook eggs an additional minute with skillet covered.
5. Slide each egg onto a plate. Pour tomato mixture onto eggs, covering each egg completely.
6. Season eggs with remaining salt and pepper, and garnish each egg with half of cilantro and jalapeño.

Per Serving: | Calories: 289 | Fat: 24.2g | Protein: 8.0g | Sodium: 469mg | Fiber: 2.4g | Carbohydrates: 9.2g | Net Carbohydrates: 6.8g | Sugar: 5.3g

Top It Off with an Avocado

Make your Huevos Rancheros a complete breakfast by serving half a sliced avocado on top of each egg. Avocados are a rich source of healthy fats: they're composed of 67 percent monosaturated fats, which support cardiovascular health.

Farmers' Scrambler

Farmers understand that a healthy breakfast is the best way to prepare for a long day of work. Starting your day strong will help you finish it strong.

* Under 500 Calories *

INGREDIENTS | SERVES 6

2 cups peeled and diced Russet potatoes
3 tablespoons olive oil, divided
½ cup sliced white mushrooms
¼ cup seeded and chopped red bell peppers
¼ cup peeled and chopped red onion
8 large eggs
¼ teaspoon salt
¼ teaspoon freshly ground black pepper

1. In a medium sauté pan, sauté potatoes in 1½ tablespoons olive oil over medium heat until tender, about 10 minutes.
2. In a separate medium sauté pan, heat remaining oil, add mushrooms, peppers, and onion and sauté over medium heat 5 minutes.
3. Combine contents of both pans in one large pan.
4. In a medium bowl, beat eggs. Add to vegetable mixture and scramble over medium heat 3 minutes.
5. Season with salt and pepper and enjoy.

Per Serving: | Calories: 193 | Fat: 11.9g | Protein: 9.5g | Sodium: 194mg | Fiber: 0.9g | Carbohydrates: 10.5g | Net Carbohydrates: 9.6g | Sugar: 1.6g

Give It a French Touch

Add 1 tablespoon of the classic French herb blend herbes de Provence to give your scrambler a little something extra. This blend usually includes savory marjoram, rosemary, thyme, oregano, and lavender. You can find this herb mixture in most supermarkets.

CHAPTER 8

Lunch

Roasted Beet Slaw

Fresh beets are versatile, flavorful, and healthy, but don't just use the root bulbs. The leafy green stalks are also good for you, and they go great in stews and salads.

* Under 500 Calories *

INGREDIENTS | SERVES 6

1 teaspoon sea salt
3 large beets, scrubbed
2 tablespoons olive oil
¼ cup balsamic vinegar
3 cups thinly sliced bitter beet greens
¼ cup raisins
1 teaspoon toasted pine nuts
¼ teaspoon salt
¼ teaspoon freshly cracked black peppercorns

1. Preheat oven to 350°F.
2. Sprinkle sea salt on an ungreased sheet pan. Toss beets in oil and place on salt bed; roast approximately 1 hour until beets are fork-tender.
3. While beets are roasting, heat vinegar in a large sauté pan over medium heat 1 minute. Add greens and raisins; heat until greens are wilted and raisins have plumped up a little, about 3 minutes.
4. Remove beets from oven and, when cool enough, peel and finely slice them. Mix together sliced beets, greens, raisins, and pine nuts in a medium bowl; season with salt and pepper and serve.

Per Serving: | Calories: 91 | Fat: 4.7g | Protein: 1.4g | Sodium: 239mg | Fiber: 2.1g | Carbohydrates: 11.4g | Net Carbohydrates: 9.3g | Sugar: 8.1g

Cooking Beets

Cook beets in their skins to prevent loss of color. This will work with any cooking method. Once cooked, the skins will slip right off!

Spicy Shrimp with Lemon Yogurt on Wilted Greens

Prepare this delicious lemon yogurt a day in advance and you will never wonder how to dress up your shrimp again!

* Under 500 Calories *

INGREDIENTS | SERVES 4

1 cup organic, grass-fed, full-fat plain yogurt
¼ cup fresh lemon zest
6 cups bitter greens
12 large shrimp (approximately ½ pound), peeled and deveined, tails on
1 teaspoon olive oil
2 cloves garlic, peeled
¼ teaspoon freshly cracked black peppercorns
¼ cup thinly sliced black olives
1 medium lemon, thinly sliced

1. Prepare yogurt sauce by mixing together yogurt and zest, then cover and refrigerate overnight.
2. Wilt greens in a steamer, about 4 minutes, then chill in the refrigerator immediately, about 10 minutes.
3. Butterfly shrimp by cutting down the center of the back almost but not completely through, then pushing down halves to form a butterfly shape.
4. In a large bowl, coat shrimp with oil, garlic, and pepper. Transfer to large skillet and cook over medium heat 5 minutes, until shrimp have turned white and pink and are firm to the touch.
5. Place greens in mounds on serving plates, then add shrimp. Dollop lemon yogurt on top of shrimp. Sprinkle each serving with olives and garnish with lemon slices.

Per Serving: | Calories: 89 | Fat: 4.3g | Protein: 6.2g | Sodium: 227mg | Fiber: 1.5g | Carbohydrates: 7.0g | Net Carbohydrates: 5.5g | Sugar: 4.6g

Traditional Greek Salad

Salads are a great way to optimize vegetable intake when following a fasting regimen. Don't be afraid to pile on any vegetables that you like to optimize your daily micronutrient intake.

* Under 500 Calories *

INGREDIENTS | SERVES 6

½ head iceberg lettuce, trimmed, cored, and torn into bite-sized pieces
½ head romaine, trimmed, cored, and torn into bite-sized pieces
1 medium red onion, peeled and sliced
1 medium cucumber, sliced
2 small beefsteak tomatoes, quartered
¼ bunch fresh oregano, chopped and stems discarded
¼ cup extra-virgin olive oil
¾ cup red wine vinegar
¼ teaspoon freshly cracked black peppercorns
6 ounces feta cheese, crumbled
2 ounces jarred pepperoncini
6 anchovy fillets
½ cup cured Greek olives

1. On a serving platter or in a large bowl, build salad by layering lettuces and vegetables.
2. In a small bowl, mix oregano with oil, vinegar, and black pepper to create dressing.
3. Drizzle dressing over salad. Top with crumbled feta, pepperoncini, anchovies, and olives.

Per Serving: | Calories: 253 | Fat: 20.4g | Protein: 7.1g | Sodium: 850mg | Fiber: 2.6g | Carbohydrates: 9.4g | Net Carbohydrates: 6.8g | Sugar: 5.1g

Carrot Thyme Soup

If your carrots are not "sweet" enough, try adding a sweet potato to the soup. Peel the potato, dice into small squares, and add to the stockpot with the other ingredients.

* Under 500 Calories *

INGREDIENTS | SERVES 6

2 pounds large carrots, peeled and diced
1 large Vidalia onion, peeled and diced
4 red potatoes, peeled and diced
3 cloves garlic, peeled and minced
1 tablespoon olive oil
6 cups vegetable stock
4 sprigs fresh thyme, stems removed
¼ teaspoon salt
¼ teaspoon freshly cracked black peppercorns

1. Place carrots, onion, potatoes, and garlic in large stockpot with oil. Sweat slowly over medium heat approximately 10 minutes.
2. Add stock and bring to a simmer; cook uncovered approximately 1 hour.
3. Remove mixture from heat and let cool slightly, about 5 minutes, then purée in a blender until smooth.
4. Return purée to pot and add thyme, salt, and pepper; cook uncovered over low heat 30 minutes. Spoon into bowls and serve.

Per Serving: | Calories: 204 | Fat: 3.5g | Protein: 5.8g | Sodium: 1,068mg | Fiber: 6.6g | Carbohydrates: 40.9g | Net Carbohydrates: 34.3g | Sugar: 9.7g

Sweating Vegetables

The term *sweat* refers to the cooking process by which the food is covered and cooked on low heat slowly until softened but not browned.

Escarole with Rich Poultry Broth

Escarole is a leafy green that's a member of the chicory family. You can also substitute endive, chicory, or kale.

* Under 500 Calories *

INGREDIENTS | SERVES 6

1 tablespoon olive oil
3 pounds skinless, bone-in chicken
2 large yellow onions, peeled and sliced
4 cloves garlic, peeled and minced
1 cup dry red wine
3 quarts no-sugar-added chicken stock
1 bunch fresh flat-leaf parsley, chopped and stems discarded
½ bunch fresh thyme, chopped and stems discarded
3 dried bay leaves
10 black peppercorns
¼ teaspoon salt
2 bunches escarole, trimmed and cored

1. Heat oil on medium heat in a medium-sized stockpot. Add chicken, onions, and garlic; sauté until chicken is golden brown, about 10 minutes.
2. Pour in wine and let reduce by half by simmering over low heat uncovered about 7 minutes. Add stock and simmer uncovered 2½ hours.
3. Add herbs and peppercorns to pot and simmer uncovered another 30 minutes. Season with salt, then strain and reserve broth. Reserve chicken on a plate to cool during next step.
4. Steam trimmed, cored escarole in a steamer approximately 5 minutes, until barely wilted. To serve, place the escarole in the bottom of serving bowls and ladle in broth.
5. Once chicken has cooled, remove and discard bones from chicken and add chicken meat to bowls of soup.

Per Serving: | Calories: 471 | Fat: 12.4g | Protein: 55.1g | Sodium: 958mg | Fiber: 5.6g | Carbohydrates: 28.8g | Net Carbohydrates: 23.2g | Sugar: 10.1g

Dandelion and White Bean Soup

Dandelions aren't just weeds—they're nutrient-rich greens that are packed with fiber, vitamin K, vitamin C, and vitamin A!

*** Under 500 Calories ***

INGREDIENTS | SERVES 6

1 teaspoon olive oil
2 medium yellow onions, peeled and chopped
3 medium carrots, peeled and diced
3 stalks celery, diced
4 cloves garlic, peeled and minced
2 quarts vegetable stock
1 dried bay leaf
¼ bunch fresh flat-leaf parsley, chopped and stems discarded
4 sprigs fresh thyme, stems discarded and leaves chopped
¼ teaspoon freshly cracked black peppercorns
2 cups fresh dandelion greens
1 cup cooked cannellini beans
¼ cup freshly grated Romano or Parmesan cheese

1. Heat oil in a large stockpot over medium heat 1 minute. Add onions, carrots, celery, and garlic; sauté until light brown, about 4 minutes.
2. Add stock and simmer on low heat uncovered 1½ hours.
3. Add herbs and spices to pot; simmer uncovered another 30 minutes.
4. Steam dandelion greens in a steamer about 7 minutes, until al dente. Add greens and beans to soup; simmer uncovered 15 minutes.
5. Ladle soup into serving bowls and sprinkle with cheese.

Per Serving: | Calories: 125 | Fat: 3.3g | Protein: 7.9g | Sodium: 1,257mg | Fiber: 4.5g | Carbohydrates: 19.2g | Net Carbohydrates: 14.7g | Sugar: 4.5g

Dandelion Greens

If you are having difficulty finding dandelion greens in your local market, try an area specialty market or farmers' market. They are a bitter yet hearty leafy vegetable. If you can't find them, you can also substitute arugula or beet greens.

Wild Rice Salad with Mushrooms and Almonds

This is a vegetarian recipe, but if you want to add some animal protein, try sautéed shrimp or diced baked chicken breast.

*** Under 500 Calories ***

INGREDIENTS | SERVES 8

¼ cup yellow raisins
1 cup filtered water
1 cup uncooked wild rice
3 cups water, lightly salted
1 cup whole raw almonds
1 tablespoon extra-virgin olive oil
8 ounces shiitake mushrooms, sliced
¼ teaspoon salt
¼ teaspoon freshly ground black pepper
2 scallions, trimmed and chopped
1 teaspoon ground cumin
Juice of 1 medium lemon (about 2 tablespoons)

1. Soak raisins in 1 cup warm water 30 minutes up to overnight.
2. Boil wild rice in a medium pot on high heat in lightly salted water until tender and most grains have burst open, about 35 minutes. Drain.
3. Lightly toast almonds in a dry small skillet over medium heat until most have small, dark brown spots and they attain an oily sheen, about 5 minutes. Spread almonds on a plate to cool, about 10 minutes, until room temperature.
4. Heat oil in a medium skillet over high heat 1 minute, then cook mushrooms until tender, about 5 minutes. Season mushrooms with salt and pepper.
5. In a mixing bowl combine rice, almonds, mushrooms (with cooking oil), raisins, and scallions. Set aside.
6. Toast cumin in dry small skillet until fragrant, about 3 minutes. Remove from heat.
7. Toss bowl of rice mixture with lemon juice and toasted cumin. Serve chilled or at room temperature.

Per Serving: | Calories: 216 | Fat: 10.4g | Protein: 7.6g | Sodium: 84mg | Fiber: 4.5g | Carbohydrates: 25.4g | Net Carbohydrates: 20.9g | Sugar: 5.1g

Warm Spinach Salad with Potatoes, Red Onions, and Kalamata Olives

Use this simple, tasty dish as a master recipe: a starting point from which to make myriad variations of your own!

* Under 500 Calories *

INGREDIENTS | SERVES 4

10 cups fresh curly leaf spinach, washed, stems removed
1 pound small red potatoes, scrubbed and cut into ½" slices
¼ cup extra-virgin olive oil
1 medium red onion, peeled, halved, and thinly sliced
20 Kalamata olives, pitted
1 tablespoon balsamic vinegar
¼ teaspoon salt
¼ teaspoon freshly ground black pepper

1. In a large mixing bowl, add spinach leaves.
2. In a medium pot, boil potatoes 10 minutes on high heat. Drain.
3. Heat olive oil in a large skillet over high heat 1 minute. Add potatoes and onion and cook until potatoes are slightly browned, about 5 minutes. Remove from heat; add olives, vinegar, salt, and pepper.
4. Pour potato mixture over spinach and invert skillet over bowl to hold in heat. Allow to steam 1 minute. Divide onto four plates, arranging potatoes, onions, and olives on top. Serve warm.

Per Serving: | Calories: **269** | Fat: 18.4g | Protein: 4.5g | Sodium: 499mg | Fiber: 4.4g | Carbohydrates: 23.0g | Net Carbohydrates: 18.6g | Sugar: 2.3g

Lentil Salad

Lentils are rich in carbohydrates, but their high fiber content slows down digestion, which can help stabilize blood sugar and energy. This tasty Lentil Salad is a great way to break your overnight fast.

* Under 500 Calories *

INGREDIENTS | SERVES 8

1 pound dried lentils, washed, undesirables discarded

2 quarts lightly salted water

2 medium yellow onions, peeled and finely chopped

3 scallions, trimmed and chopped

1 medium green bell pepper, stemmed, seeded, and finely chopped

1 tablespoon cumin powder

⅛ teaspoon cayenne pepper

Juice of 1 medium lemon (about ¼ cup)

2 tablespoons extra-virgin olive oil

¼ teaspoon salt

¼ teaspoon freshly ground black pepper

1. Boil lentils in a medium pot with water on high heat until tender but not broken up, about 12 minutes. Spread on a pan to cool 5 minutes.
2. In a large bowl, combine lentils with onions, scallions, and green pepper.
3. Toast cumin in small dry skillet until fragrant, about 3 minutes. Remove from heat.
4. Toss cumin and remaining ingredients in bowl with lentil mixture and serve.

Per Serving: | Calories: 211 | Fat: 3.9g | Protein: 13.6g | Sodium: 417mg | Fiber: 12.2g | Carbohydrates: 32.1g | Net Carbohydrates: 19.9g | Sugar: 4.3g

California Garden Salad with Avocado and Sprouts

The fruity taste of large green Florida avocados gives this salad a lighter, more summery flavor than the original California Hass avocado.

* Under 500 Calories *

INGREDIENTS | SERVES 4

Dressing

1 tablespoon freshly squeezed lemon juice

3 tablespoons extra-virgin olive oil

1 tablespoon finely chopped shallot

½ teaspoon salt

¼ teaspoon freshly ground black pepper

Salad

2 heads Boston or Bibb lettuce, trimmed and cored

2 large ripe beefsteak tomatoes, cored and cut into 8 wedges each

1 ripe medium avocado, peeled, pitted, and cut into 8 wedges

1 cup alfalfa sprouts

1. **To make dressing:** combine lemon juice, olive oil, shallot, salt, and pepper in a small bowl, mixing well.
2. **To make salad:** arrange lettuce leaves, stem ends in, onto four plates, making a flower petal pattern. Inner leaves will be too small, so reserve them for another use.
3. Toss tomatoes in 1 tablespoon dressing; place 4 tomato wedges on each salad. Toss avocado with another 1 tablespoon dressing; place 2 avocado wedges on each salad. Divide sprouts among plates. Drizzle salads with remaining dressing or serve it on the side.

Per Serving: | Calories: 179 | Fat: 14.8g | Protein: 3.1g | Sodium: 302mg | Fiber: 4.7g | Carbohydrates: 9.7g | Net Carbohydrates: 5.0g | Sugar: 3.8g

Pumpkin Soup with Caraway Seeds

Butternut squash, or even acorn squash, substitutes very well for pumpkin in this soup. Each imparts its own character, making this three recipes in one. Chipotle or Spanish paprika (both found in gourmet stores) add a subtle smokiness for an additional flavor dimension.

* Under 500 Calories *

INGREDIENTS | SERVES 8

2 tablespoons unsalted grass-fed butter
1 medium yellow onion, peeled and chopped
1 large carrot, peeled and thinly sliced
2 cups peeled and cubed pumpkin
¼ teaspoon whole caraway seeds
1½ cups vegetable stock
3 cups unsweetened full-fat coconut milk, divided
¼ teaspoon salt
¼ teaspoon freshly ground black pepper
½ teaspoon dried chipotle chili pepper

1. Melt butter in a large, heavy-bottomed soup pot over medium heat 1 minute. Add onion, carrot, pumpkin, and caraway seeds; sauté, stirring occasionally, 10 minutes until pumpkin becomes tender and begins to brown (some may stick to pan).
2. Add stock and simmer covered 20 minutes. Remove from heat and stir in 2 cups milk.
3. Purée soup in batches in a blender until smooth, adjusting consistency with remaining milk. Season with salt and pepper. Sprinkle chipotle chili pepper or Spanish paprika on top for garnish.

Per Serving: | Calories: 214 | Fat: 20.0g | Protein: 2.3g | Sodium: 200mg | Fiber: 0.9g | Carbohydrates: 7.1g | Net Carbohydrates: 6.2g | Sugar: 2.0g

Using Smoked Chilies or Spices to Add Smoky Flavor

For a smoky flavor, nonvegetarian recipes often call for smoked pork bones or bacon. Vegetarians can achieve a similar result by adding smoked whole chilies, such as chipotle (smoked jalapeño) to dishes.

Smooth Cauliflower Soup with Coriander

Because this soup is puréed, it's easy on digestion. Eating this creamy dish as your first meal after your fasting window will help slowly kick on your digestion and ease your body into the day.

*** Under 500 Calories ***

INGREDIENTS | SERVES 4

2 tablespoons unsalted grass-fed butter

1 medium yellow onion, peeled and diced

2 tablespoons white wine

1 large head (about 2 pounds) cauliflower, cored and cut into bite-sized pieces

2 cups vegetable stock

1 teaspoon salt

¼ teaspoon ground white pepper

1 teaspoon ground coriander

¾ cup unsweetened full-fat coconut milk, divided

¼ teaspoon chopped fresh chives

1. In a large saucepan or soup pot, melt butter over medium-high heat 1 minute. Add onion; cook about 5 minutes until translucent but not brown.
2. Add wine and cauliflower; cook 1 minute to steam out alcohol. Add the stock, salt, pepper, and coriander; bring to a rolling boil over high heat, then turn heat to low.
3. Let mixture simmer until cauliflower is very tender, about 15 minutes. Transfer to a blender. Add half of milk and purée until very smooth, scraping down the sides of the blender with a rubber spatula. Be very careful during this step, as hot liquids will splash out of blender if not started gradually (you may want to purée in two batches, for safety).
4. Transfer soup back to saucepan and thin with additional milk if desired. Garnish with chopped herbs just before serving.

Per Serving: | Calories: 214 | Fat: 15.5g | Protein: 6.4g | Sodium: 1,100mg | Fiber: 4.9g | Carbohydrates: 15.5g | Net Carbohydrates: 10.6g | Sugar: 5.6g

Vichyssoise (Potato and Leek Soup)

Comforting and easy to prepare, this soup will leave you full and satisfied. If you are incorporating a low-carbohydrate diet into your fasting plan, you can adjust this recipe by using turnips in place of potatoes. Replace the potatoes with equal amounts of turnips and cook the same way.

* Under 500 Calories *

INGREDIENTS | SERVES 12

1 tablespoon olive oil
1 medium yellow onion, peeled and chopped
1 pound (about 4 medium) potatoes, any variety, peeled and cut into 1" chunks
2 bunches leeks, washed twice, chopped, and divided
1 teaspoon dried sage
1 bay leaf
¼ cup white wine
2 quarts vegetable stock
¼ teaspoon salt
¼ teaspoon ground white pepper

1. In a large soup pot over medium heat, heat olive oil 1 minute. Add onion, potatoes, and all but 1 bunch leeks; cook 10 minutes, until onions are translucent. Add sage, bay leaf, and wine. Cook an additional minute.
2. Add stock to pot. Bring to a full boil on high heat, then reduce heat to low and cook 45 minutes until potatoes are very tender and starting to fall apart.
3. Carefully purée soup in a blender in small batches. Season with salt and white pepper.
4. Steam, boil, or sauté remaining 1 bunch leeks, about 4 minutes, and serve soup garnished with a spoonful of leeks in the center of each bowl.

Per Serving: | Calories: 101 | Fat: 1.9g | Protein: 3.2g | Sodium: 628mg | Fiber: 2.0g | Carbohydrates: 19.5g | Net Carbohydrates: 17.5g | Sugar: 3.1g

Chickpeas in Potato Onion Curry

Thirty-minute main dishes like this are a lifesaver when you come home hungry and nothing's ready for dinner. Before you start this dish, put on a pot of brown rice to serve with it and you'll be dining before you know it.

* Under 500 Calories *

INGREDIENTS | SERVES 4

2 large yellow onions, peeled and cut into 1" pieces
3 tablespoons olive oil, divided
1½ cups peeled and cubed (1" pieces) Russet potatoes
1 (13.5-ounce) can unsweetened full-fat coconut milk
1 (15-ounce) can chickpeas (garbanzo beans), drained and rinsed
6 cloves garlic, peeled
1 teaspoon salt
1½ teaspoons ground coriander
½ teaspoon ground turmeric
1 teaspoon chili powder
1 teaspoon ground cumin
Juice of ½ medium lemon

1. In a large skillet over high heat, cook onions in 1 tablespoon oil until lightly browned, about 5 minutes. Add potatoes and milk; cover and cook until potatoes are tender, about 20 minutes. Add chickpeas and reduce heat to low.
2. In a food processor, combine garlic, salt, coriander, turmeric, chili powder, and cumin; process until mixture becomes a paste, scraping down sides of processor as needed.
3. Heat remaining oil in a small skillet and fry paste 1 minute until fragrant and slightly browned.
4. Add cooked paste to potato mixture. Simmer 3 minutes. Season with lemon juice and serve.

Per Serving: | Calories: 451 | Fat: 30.5g | Protein: 8.7g | Sodium: 754mg | Fiber: 6.7g | Carbohydrates: 37.0g | Net Carbohydrates: 30.3g | Sugar: 6.7g

Red Pepper Soup

The few drops of vanilla enhance the savory flavors of this delightful soup. Serve it warm in winter—sans the toppings—or cool, as described, in the summer months.

* Under 500 Calories *

INGREDIENTS | SERVES 6

1 tablespoon olive oil

3 medium red bell peppers, stemmed, seeded, and diced

1 large red potato, peeled and diced

1 cup peeled and diced carrots

1 large parsnip, peeled and diced

6 cups water

¼ teaspoon sea salt

⅛ teaspoon freshly ground black pepper

⅛ teaspoon alcohol-free vanilla extract

¾ cup canned unsweetened full-fat coconut milk, refrigerated

¼ cup chopped fresh chives, divided

1. Heat oil over medium-low heat in a large stockpot 1 minute.
2. Add vegetables to pot and sauté 10 minutes. Add water. Bring to a boil on high heat, then turn heat to low and simmer uncovered 3 hours until vegetables are very tender. Season with salt and pepper. Stir in vanilla. Remove from heat and let cool completely, about 15 minutes.
3. Once cool, purée soup in batches in a food processor or blender until completely smooth.
4. Divide soup into six individual serving bowls. Swirl 2 tablespoons milk into each bowl and sprinkle with chives.

Per Serving: | Calories: 162 | Fat: 8.0g | Protein: 2.6g | Sodium: 90mg | Fiber: 3.9g | Carbohydrates: 20.6g | Net Carbohydrates: 16.7g | Sugar: 5.1g

Chicken Piccata

This lunchtime (or anytime!) treat is a great blend of protein, zesty lemon, and artichokes.

*** Under 500 Calories ***

INGREDIENTS | SERVES 4

1 cup no-salt-added chicken broth
½ cup freshly squeezed lemon juice
4 skinless, boneless chicken breasts
3 tablespoons olive oil
1 cup chopped yellow onion
1 clove garlic, minced
2 cups chopped fresh artichoke hearts
3 tablespoons capers
1 teaspoon pepper

1. Combine chicken broth, lemon juice, and chicken in shallow dish. Cover and marinate overnight in the refrigerator.
2. Heat olive oil 30 seconds in a medium sauté pan over medium heat, then add onion and garlic and cook until softened, about 2 minutes.
3. Remove chicken from marinade, reserving marinade. Add chicken to pan and brown on each side, 8 minutes total.
4. Add artichoke hearts, capers, pepper, and reserved marinade. Reduce heat to low and simmer until chicken is thoroughly cooked, about 10 minutes.

Per Serving: | Calories: 295 | Fat: 12.3g | Protein: 30.1g | Sodium: 307mg | Fiber: 5.2g | Carbohydrates: 14.8g | Net Carbohydrates: 9.6g | Sugar: 3.3g

Capers

Capers are salted and should be used only occasionally for a dish such as this one where they are integral to a favorite recipe. If you aren't a fan, this dish is still full of flavor without them.

Shredded Chicken Wraps

Lettuce wraps are a great way to get the feel of a tortilla wrap without the carbohydrates. You can easily substitute your favorite meat or fish for the chicken to vary your menu.

* Under 500 Calories *

INGREDIENTS | SERVES 8

2 boneless, skinless chicken breasts, baked and shredded
2 stalks celery, chopped
¼ cup chopped fresh basil
2 tablespoons olive oil
2 tablespoons freshly squeezed lemon juice
1 teaspoon peeled minced garlic
⅛ teaspoon freshly ground black pepper
1 head radicchio

1. Mix chicken in a large bowl with celery, basil, olive oil, lemon juice, garlic, and pepper.
2. Separate radicchio lettuce leaves and place on 8 plates.
3. Spoon chicken mixture onto lettuce leaves and roll up.

Per Serving: | Calories: 68 | Fat: 3.4g | Protein: 6.6g | Sodium: 22mg | Fiber: 0.3g | Carbohydrates: 1.1g | Net Carbohydrates: 0.8g | Sugar: 0.3g

Curried Chicken Salad

This recipe makes two servings, but you can double or triple the ingredient amounts for a family gathering. You can also change the spices around for more variety.

* Under 500 Calories *

INGREDIENTS | SERVES 2

2 tablespoons olive oil
8 ounces boneless, skinless chicken breast, cubed
1 stalk celery, sliced
1 small yellow onion, diced
½ English cucumber, diced
½ cup chopped raw almonds
2 medium apples, chopped
½ teaspoon curry powder
4 cups baby romaine lettuce

1. In large sauté pan over medium heat, cook chicken, celery, and onion thoroughly in olive oil 10 minutes. Set aside to cool 15 minutes.
2. In a large mixing bowl combine cucumber, almonds, apples, and curry powder with cooled chicken mixture.
3. Serve over bed of baby romaine lettuce.

Per Serving: | Calories: 124 | Fat: 6.6g | Protein: 8.2g | Sodium: 19mg | Fiber: 2.4g | Carbohydrates: 8.1g | Net Carbohydrates: 5.7g | Sugar: 4.5g

Cage Free

Cage-free, barn-roaming chickens are an important component of a healthy diet. Chickens raised in commercial chicken farms are fed a corn-based diet with low omega-3 fatty acid content. Additionally, they are kept in coops where they get little exercise and are fed antibiotics to maintain their health—antibiotics that will filter into your food.

Chicken with Sautéed Tomatoes and Pine Nuts

Sautéed tomatoes and pine nuts add a nice, nutty flavor to an ordinary dish. This topping can also be added to fish or beef.

⋆ Under 500 Calories ⋆

INGREDIENTS | SERVES 4

¼ cup olive oil
1 cup halved cherry tomatoes
¼ cup green chilies, chopped
¼ cup fresh cilantro
½ cup pine nuts
2 boneless skinless chicken breasts

1. Heat olive oil 30 seconds in a medium skillet over medium-high heat. Sauté tomatoes, chilies, cilantro, and pine nuts until golden brown, about 5 minutes. Set aside.
2. In the same pan, cook chicken 5 minutes on each side.
3. Return tomato mixture to pan and cover. Simmer on low 5 minutes until chicken is fully cooked.

Per Serving: | Calories: 311 | Fat: 23.9g | Protein: 15.6g | Sodium: 28mg | Fiber: 1.2g | Carbohydrates: 4.6g | Net Carbohydrates: 3.4g | Sugar: 2.1g

Butter Lettuce Salad with Poached Eggs and Bacon

This Butter Lettuce Salad with Poached Eggs and Bacon is the perfect light lunch to eat during your feeding window. It contains plenty of protein to keep you full but won't weigh you down after fasting.

* Under 500 Calories *

INGREDIENTS | SERVES 4

4 slices thick-cut, no-sugar-added nitrate-free bacon
1 tablespoon freshly squeezed lemon juice
2 teaspoons Dijon mustard
2 tablespoons extra-virgin olive oil
½ teaspoon freshly ground black pepper
3 cups water
1 tablespoon rice wine vinegar
4 large eggs
4 cups butter lettuce leaves

1. Preheat oven to 400°F.
2. Line a rimmed baking sheet with parchment paper and place bacon on top of paper. Bake 18 minutes until crisp and browned, rotating baking sheet once halfway through. Drain bacon strips on a paper towel–lined plate. Let cool 5 minutes. Once cool enough to handle, cut bacon into ½" pieces.
3. In a small bowl, combine lemon juice, mustard, oil, and pepper. Stir well to combine.
4. Pour cold water into a large saucepan until there is at least 4" water. Add vinegar and bring to a boil over medium heat, then reduce heat to low.
5. In a small shallow bowl, crack 1 egg. Stir water in saucepan continuously to create a whirlpool. Gently pour egg into water. Cook egg 4 minutes until firm. Remove from water with a slotted spoon. Skim any remaining foam from water. Repeat with remaining eggs.
6. In a large salad bowl, add lettuce and bacon. Pour on lemon-mustard dressing. Toss well to combine. Divide among four plates. Gently add one egg to each plate and serve.

Per Serving: | Calories: 198 | Fat: 15.1g | Protein: 11.2g | Sodium: 329mg | Fiber: 0.7g | Carbohydrates: 2.4g | Net Carbohydrates: 1.7g | Sugar: 0.8g

Zesty Pecan, Chicken, and Grape Salad

Coating your chicken with nuts adds a crispy skin to keep the breast inside moist and tender.

⋆ Under 500 Calories ⋆

INGREDIENTS | SERVES 6

¼ cup chopped pecans
1 teaspoon chili powder
¼ cup extra-virgin olive oil
6 boneless, skinless chicken breasts (about 1½ pounds)
6 cups salad greens, torn into bite-sized pieces
1½ cups sliced white grapes

1. Preheat oven to 400°F.
2. In a blender, mix chopped nuts and chili powder. Pour in oil while blender is running. When mixture is thoroughly combined, pour into a shallow bowl.
3. Coat chicken with pecan mixture and place on rack in a 9" × 13" ungreased baking dish. Roast 50 minutes until chicken is thoroughly cooked. Remove from oven, let cool 5 minutes, then thinly slice.
4. To serve, fan chicken over greens on six plates and sprinkle with sliced grapes.

Per Serving: | Calories: 279 | Fat: 13.9g | Protein: 26.6g | Sodium: 88mg | Fiber: 1.6g | Carbohydrate: 8.7g | Net Carbohydrates: 7.1g | Sugar: 6.2g

Toasting Nuts for Fresher Flavor and Crispness

To wake the natural flavor of nuts, heat them on the stovetop or in the oven for a few minutes. On the stovetop, spread nuts in a dry skillet and heat over a medium flame until their natural oils come to the surface. In the oven, spread the nuts in a single layer on an ungreased baking sheet and toast 5–10 minutes at 350°F until the oils are visible.

Curried Shrimp with Vegetables

This recipe is delicious as written and also easy to adapt with whatever you have on hand to make preparation even easier. You can swap the shrimp for chicken or beef and use any vegetables that you like.

* Under 500 Calories *

INGREDIENTS | SERVES 4

2 tablespoons olive oil

1 tablespoon green curry powder

1 pound shrimp, peeled and deveined

1 (12-ounce) bag frozen broccoli florets

4 large carrots, peeled and sliced

1 (8-ounce) can unsweetened full-fat coconut milk

1. In a large skillet over medium heat, warm olive oil and green curry powder 1 minute.
2. Add shrimp, broccoli, carrots, and milk to skillet. Cook until vegetables are tender and milk has a thick, pastelike consistency, approximately 15 minutes. Serve warm.

Per Serving: | Calories: 310 | Fat: 19.2g | Protein: 20.1g | Sodium: 815mg | Fiber: 4.7g | Carbohydrate: 14.8g | Net Carbohydrates: 10.1g | Sugar: 4.8g

Turkey Meatballs

This is an easy meatball recipe with a few delicious additions. You can substitute any type of ground meat, including bison, beef, chicken, or pork. And flaxseed meal can replace the almond meal.

* Under 500 Calories *

INGREDIENTS | SERVES 8

2 pounds 85 percent lean ground turkey
1 cup almond meal
2 large eggs
5 scallions, trimmed and chopped
1 medium red bell pepper, stemmed, seeded, and diced
2 cloves garlic, peeled and minced
1 tablespoon dried basil
1 tablespoon dried oregano
2 tablespoons olive oil

1. Preheat oven to 400°F.
2. In a large bowl, combine all ingredients except olive oil. Mix well with clean hands.
3. Add olive oil to turkey mixture and mix well.
4. Form turkey mixture into 24 meatballs and place on two rimmed ungreased baking pans.
5. Bake 20 minutes. Serve warm.

Per Serving: | Calories: 351 | Fat: 24.2g | Protein: 26.1g | Sodium: 84mg | Fiber: 2.2g | Carbohydrate: 4.8g | Net Carbohydrates: 2.6g | Sugar: 1.3g

Higher-Fat Ground Meats

Although most people make sure to buy the lowest-fat ground meat, it is more beneficial to buy fattier ground meat when it is from grass-fed or barn-roaming animals. This meat is lower in saturated fat than most commercial ground meat and contains more omega-3 fatty acids.

Coconut-Crumbed Chicken

Coconut is an easy way to add some flavor and crunch to chicken (or firm fish and shrimp!) while keeping the recipe gluten-free.

* Under 500 Calories *

INGREDIENTS | SERVES 8

1 cup ground almond meal
2 large eggs
2 teaspoons freshly ground black pepper
1 tablespoon Italian seasoning
1 cup ground unsweetened shredded coconut
½ cup flaxseed meal
16 chicken tenderloins (approximately 2 pounds)
4 tablespoons coconut oil

1. In a small shallow bowl, add almond meal. In another bowl, whisk together eggs, pepper, and Italian seasoning. In a third bowl, combine coconut with flaxseed meal.
2. Coat chicken pieces first in almond meal, then egg mixture, then coconut mixture.
3. Heat coconut oil in a large nonstick skillet over medium-high heat, about 1 minute. Pan-fry tenderloins in skillet until cooked through, approximately 5 minutes on each side.
4. Transfer chicken to plates and serve.

Per Serving: | Calories: 353 | Fat: 23.2g | Protein: 27.6g | Sodium: 121mg | Fiber: 5.2g | Carbohydrate: 8.1g | Net Carbohydrates: 2.9g | Sugar: 1.2g

Paleo Stuffed Peppers

Peppers are chock-full of great vitamins and minerals that everyone needs, and they also provide a great base for filling. You can adapt this basic recipe to use whatever ingredients you have on hand.

* Under 500 Calories *

INGREDIENTS | SERVES 4

2 tablespoons olive oil
3 cloves garlic, peeled and chopped
1 large yellow onion, peeled and chopped
1 pound ground chicken
2 medium green bell peppers, stemmed, seeded, and chopped
1 cup diced celery
1 cup sliced white mushrooms
2 tablespoons chili powder
1 tablespoon ground cumin
4 medium red bell peppers, tops cut off, seeds and ribs removed
1 (28-ounce) can organic, no-salt-added diced tomatoes, drained
1 (6-ounce) can organic, no-salt-added tomato paste

1. In large skillet, heat olive oil over medium heat 1 minute, then sauté garlic and onion 2 minutes.
2. Add ground chicken and cook until browned, about 5 minutes. Add green peppers, celery, mushrooms, chili powder, and cumin and continue cooking 5 minutes.
3. Stuff mixture into red peppers and place in slow cooker.
4. Combine diced tomatoes and tomato paste and pour over peppers; cook on high 5 hours.

Per Serving: | Calories: 397 | Fat: 16.5g | Protein: 26.8g | Sodium: 274mg | Fiber: 10.3g | Carbohydrate: 35.8g | Net Carbohydrates: 25.5g | Sugar: 18.5g

South American Chili

This makes a great hot lunch on cold winter days. Make a large batch and store the extra in the refrigerator for later meals. You can even use it as a sauce over spaghetti squash.

* Under 500 Calories *

INGREDIENTS | SERVES 8

2 tablespoons olive oil
2 cups peeled and chopped yellow onions
2 cups seeded and chopped red bell peppers
4 cloves garlic, peeled and minced
2 pounds 85 percent lean ground beef
1 tablespoon ground cumin
1 teaspoon cayenne pepper
2½ tablespoons beef broth
1 cup diced vine-ripened tomatoes
½ tablespoon salt

1. Heat oil in a large pot over medium-high heat 1 minute. Add onions, peppers, and garlic and sauté 5 minutes.
2. Add ground beef, cumin, and cayenne pepper to pot. Sauté until ground beef is brown, about 8 minutes, breaking up beef with the back of a fork while cooking.
3. Add beef broth and tomatoes and reduce heat to low. Simmer until chili is thick, about 20 minutes, stirring occasionally while simmering.
4. Season with salt and ladle into bowls.

Per Serving: | Calories: 310 | Fat: 17.9g | Protein: 22.4g | Sodium: 533mg | Fiber: 1.9g | Carbohydrates: 7.8g | Net Carbohydrates: 5.9g | Sugar: 3.9g

Chicken Soup with Asparagus

The curative powers of chicken soup and asparagus join to make a warm and tasty powerhouse dish. Asparagus has high levels of folate, which can help keep the mind sharp, so this soup is a smart choice.

* Under 500 Calories *

INGREDIENTS | SERVES 6

7 cups chicken stock

2 chicken breast halves (about ½ pound each), bone-in

¾ pound asparagus spears, trimmed and cut into 1½" pieces

4 cups lightly packed, thinly sliced fresh Swiss chard leaves

4 medium plum tomatoes, seeded and chopped

½ teaspoon sea salt

½ teaspoon freshly ground black pepper

1. In a 4-quart Dutch oven, combine chicken stock and chicken. Bring to a boil over high heat, then reduce the heat to low. Simmer covered 20 minutes until the chicken is no longer pink.
2. Remove chicken from the broth; cool slightly, about 5 minutes. Discard skin and bones. Shred chicken into bite-sized pieces with two forks.
3. Add asparagus to broth and cook 3 minutes. Stir in Swiss chard, tomatoes, and shredded cooked chicken. Heat through, about 5 minutes.
4. Add salt and pepper and serve.

Per Serving: | Calories: 190 | Fat: 4.6g | Protein: 23.1g | Sodium: 605mg | Fiber: 1.6g | Carbohydrates: 13.7g | Net Carbohydrates: 12.1g | Sugar: 6.4g

Add Some Variety

Use your favorite vegetables for this recipe. Try replacing the chard with spinach, kale, or collard greens. Adding some cubed zucchini toward the end of the cooking process also gives the soup a little more texture.

Tarragon Lemon Chicken

Tarragon has been nicknamed the "King of Herbs" because its benefits go far beyond flavoring your food. Tarragon may help alleviate digestive symptoms and balance your appetite, something that can be especially helpful when you're first adjusting to fasting.

* Under 500 Calories *

INGREDIENTS | SERVES 4

⅓ cup olive oil
2 tablespoons finely chopped fresh chives
1 tablespoon finely chopped fresh cilantro
1 tablespoon freshly squeezed lemon juice
1½ teaspoons dried tarragon, crushed
¼ teaspoon paprika
4 (4-ounce) boneless, skinless chicken thighs
¼ teaspoon freshly ground black pepper

1. Place olive oil in a medium saucepan over low heat. Add chives, cilantro, lemon juice, tarragon, and paprika and stir 1 minute.
2. Season chicken with pepper and add to saucepan. Cook over medium heat in olive oil marinade until tender and no longer pink in the center, approximately 15 minutes. Serve hot or cold.

Per Serving: | Calories: 255 | Fat: 13.8g | Protein: 28.8g | Sodium: 122mg | Fiber: 0.1g | Carbohydrates: 0.1g | Net Carbohydrates: 0.0g | Sugar: 0.0g

Baked Meatballs

Baking meatballs instead of frying them saves time and cleanup, and they can easily be added to homemade tomato sauce.

* Under 500 Calories *

INGREDIENTS | SERVES 8

1½ pounds lean (85 percent or higher) ground beef
2 large eggs
½ teaspoon dried ground oregano
½ teaspoon salt
¼ teaspoon freshly ground black pepper
2 tablespoons olive oil

1. Preheat oven to 350°F.
2. In a large bowl, mix ground beef, eggs, oregano, salt, and pepper with your hands.
3. Form mixture into 16 golf ball–sized meatballs.
4. Grease a jelly roll pan with olive oil, and arrange meatballs on pan. Bake 25 minutes until meatballs are browned and cooked through.

Per Serving: | Calories: 171 | Fat: 9.8g | Protein: 16.2g | Sodium: 210mg | Fiber: 0.0g | Carbohydrates: 0.2g | Net Carbohydrates: 0.2g | Sugar: 0.1g

Gluten-Free Spaghetti and Meatballs

Make your favorite marinara or tomato sauce in a large saucepan, add the meatballs to the sauce, and let them cook 10 minutes over medium heat. Bake a medium-sized spaghetti squash for about 45 minutes. Once the squash is fully cooked, scrape the flesh out and season it with a little olive oil, salt, and pepper. Serve the spaghetti squash warm with the meatballs and tomato sauce on top.

Picadillo

Picadillo is a traditional hashlike dish originating in Latin countries and often served over rice. You can add more variety with jalapeños, olives, capers, cinnamon, cloves, or oregano.

INGREDIENTS | SERVES 4

1 tablespoon olive oil

1 pound lean (85 percent or higher) ground beef

½ cup peeled and diced yellow onion

½ cup seeded and diced green bell pepper

1 tablespoon peeled and finely minced garlic

1 teaspoon salt

1 teaspoon freshly ground black pepper

1 teaspoon ground cumin

2 large Russet potatoes, peeled and diced

2 large vine-ripened tomatoes, peeled and diced

1. Add oil to a large skillet and cook beef 5 minutes on medium heat. Add onion, bell pepper, garlic, salt, black pepper, and cumin. Continue cooking 8 minutes.
2. Add diced potatoes. Cover, lower heat, and simmer 45 minutes. Add tomatoes and simmer an additional 5 minutes.
3. Remove from heat and serve.

Per Serving: | Calories: 538 | Fat: 14.4g | Protein: 27.1g | Sodium: 656mg | Fiber: 6.7g | Carbohydrates: 70.2g | Net Carbohydrates: 63.5g | Sugar: 5.1g

CHAPTER 9

Dinner

Lamb Patties

The lamb can be served rare to medium-rare, but the egg should be thoroughly cooked. Fruit chutneys or chia seed jams are perfect complements to meat patties.

* Under 500 Calories *

INGREDIENTS | SERVES 2

1 medium shallot, peeled and minced
2 cloves garlic, peeled and minced
½ pound ground lamb
1 egg white
¼ cup dried currants
¼ cup whole pistachio nuts
½ teaspoon ground cinnamon
¼ teaspoon freshly cracked black peppercorns
⅛ teaspoon salt

1. Preheat oven to 350°F.
2. Mix shallots and garlic with lamb, egg, currants, nuts, and cinnamon. Season with pepper and salt.
3. Form mixture into 6 small ovals. Place in an 8" × 8" baking dish and bake 15 minutes. Serve warm.

Per Serving: | Calories: 399 | Fat: 21.8g | Protein: 27.3g | Sodium: 243mg | Fiber: 3.6g | Carbohydrates: 21.4g | Net Carbohydrates: 17.8g | Sugar: 14.3g

Lentil-Stuffed Peppers

These Lentil-Stuffed Peppers are even better as leftovers. Make them in advance and store them in your refrigerator for a quick meal that's ready to eat when you're ready to break your fast.

* Under 500 Calories *

INGREDIENTS | SERVES 6

1 tablespoon olive oil
2 medium yellow onions, peeled and finely diced
2 stalks celery, finely diced
2 large carrots, peeled and finely diced
4 cups vegetable stock, divided
3 cups dried red lentils
6 medium red bell peppers, tops cut off and set aside, seeds and ribs removed
6 sprigs fresh oregano, tops reserved and remaining leaves chopped
3 ounces feta cheese
¼ teaspoon freshly cracked black peppercorns

1. Heat oil in a large saucepot over medium heat 1 minute. Add onions, celery, and carrots; sauté 5 minutes, then add 1 cup vegetable stock and lentils. Simmer 20 minutes until lentils are fully cooked.
2. Place bell peppers in a large, shallow pot with 3 cups vegetable stock. Cover and simmer 10 minutes, then remove from heat.
3. In a bowl, mix together lentil mixture, oregano, feta, and black pepper; spoon mixture into bell peppers.
4. Serve peppers with stem tops ajar. Garnish with reserved oregano tops.

Per Serving: | Calories: 473 | Fat: 7.8g | Protein: 28.3g | Sodium: 745mg | Fiber: 14.3g | Carbohydrates: 75.3g | Net Carbohydrates: 61g | Sugar: 8.7g

Marinated London Broil

Cinnamon and cloves may not be your first thought when it comes to steak rubs, but these spices bring out mouthwatering flavors. After cooking, cut the London broil against the grain.

* Under 500 Calories *

INGREDIENTS | SERVES 6

1 cup dry red wine
1 tablespoon olive oil
1 teaspoon ground cinnamon
½ teaspoon ground cloves
1 teaspoon ground cumin
¼ teaspoon freshly cracked black peppercorns
¼ teaspoon salt
1½ pounds London broil

1. Preheat grill to medium heat.
2. Mix together wine, oil, and seasonings. Coat meat in mixture, then grill to desired doneness. Slice and serve.

Per Serving: | Calories: 170 | Fat: 5.7g | Protein: 24.6g | Sodium: 159mg | Fiber: 0.4g | Carbohydrates: 1.0g | Net Carbohydrates: 0.6g | Sugar: 0.1g

Smoky Black-Eyed Pea Soup with Sweet Potatoes and Mustard Greens

Black-eyed peas offer the delicious earthiness of green peas but with a savory touch. Use any dark leafy greens you'd like, fresh or frozen, in place of the mustard greens. Julienned kale or collard greens are excellent choices and are equally rich in antioxidants.

* Under 500 Calories *

INGREDIENTS | SERVES 10

1 tablespoon olive oil
1 medium yellow onion, peeled and chopped
2 stalks celery, chopped
1 large carrot, peeled and chopped
2 teaspoons salt
1 teaspoon dried thyme
2 teaspoons dried oregano
1 teaspoon ground cumin
1 dried chipotle chili, halved
2 bay leaves
1 pound dried black-eyed peas, washed and picked through for undesirables
2 quarts vegetable stock
1 large sweet potato, peeled and diced into 1" cubes
1 (10-ounce) package frozen mustard greens, chopped
1 (22-ounce) can diced tomatoes, drained
¼ teaspoon chopped fresh cilantro

1. In a large, heavy-bottomed Dutch oven, heat oil 1 minute over medium heat. Add onion, celery, carrot, and salt; cook 5 minutes until onions are translucent. Add thyme, oregano, cumin, chipotle chili, and bay leaves; cook additional 2 minutes.
2. Add black-eyed peas and vegetable stock. Bring to a boil over high heat, then simmer on low heat 2 hours, until beans are very tender.
3. Add sweet potato and cook 20 minutes. Stir in chopped mustard greens and tomatoes. Cook additional 10 minutes, until potatoes and greens are tender. Adjust consistency with additional vegetable stock. The soup should have lots of broth.
4. Serve garnished with chopped cilantro.

Per Serving: | Calories: 107 | Fat: 2.4g | Protein: 4.8g | Sodium: 1,283mg | Fiber: 5.2g | Carbohydrates: 18.6g | Net Carbohydrates: 13.4g | Sugar: 5.2g

Lentil Soup with Cumin

Ready in an hour, this is the fastest bean soup you can make. It gets better as it sits overnight, when the flavors marry, so make enough for two or more meals!

*** Under 500 Calories ***

INGREDIENTS | SERVES 8

½ teaspoon whole cumin seeds
1 tablespoon olive oil
1 large carrot, peeled and chopped
1 stalk celery, chopped
1 medium yellow onion, peeled and chopped
1 large Russet potato, peeled and chopped
2 cloves garlic, peeled and sliced
2 teaspoons salt
1 cup dried lentils
2 quarts vegetable stock

1. Toast cumin seeds in a small dry pan 1 minute until fragrant.
2. Heat oil over medium heat in a large pot 1 minute. Add vegetables, garlic, cumin, and salt. Cook 5 minutes.
3. Add lentils and vegetable stock. Raise heat to high to bring soup to a boil, then reduce heat to medium-low. Simmer 1 hour.
4. Serve warm.

Per Serving: | Calories: 146 | Fat: 3.2g | Protein: 8.6g | Sodium: 1,458mg | Fiber: 3.5g | Carbohydrates: 23.6g | Net Carbohydrates: 20.1g | Sugar: 2.1g

Tuscan White Bean Soup

Beans are full of fiber, which not only keeps you regular but also keeps you full longer. This delicious Tuscan White Bean Soup will keep your hunger at bay.

* Under 500 Calories *

INGREDIENTS | SERVES 8

2 tablespoons extra-virgin olive oil, divided
1 medium yellow onion, peeled and chopped
1 large leek, white part only, finely chopped
3 cloves garlic, peeled and finely chopped
3 teaspoons fresh chopped rosemary
1 bay leaf
3 quarts vegetable stock
2 cups large white beans (soaked overnight if desired)
¼ teaspoon salt
¼ teaspoon ground white pepper

1. In a large soup pot over medium heat, heat 1 tablespoon olive oil 1 minute. Add onion, leeks, and garlic; cook 10 minutes until onions are translucent, stirring frequently. Add rosemary and bay leaf; cook an additional 5 minutes.
2. Add stock and beans to pot. Bring to a full boil over high heat. Reduce heat to low, and cook 90 minutes until beans are very tender and starting to fall apart. Cooking time will vary depending on age of beans and whether or not they were soaked; assume 30 minutes less for soaked beans.
3. Purée ⅔ of soup in a blender; add back to rest of soup. Season with salt and pepper.
4. Serve each bowl with a few drops of extra-virgin olive oil sprinkled on top.

Per Serving: | Calories: 237 | Fat: 5.1g | Protein: 15.4g | Sodium: 1,379mg | Fiber: 8.2g | Carbohydrates: 36.3g | Net Carbohydrates: 28.1g | Sugar: 3.2g

Soaking Beans—What It Means

Some chefs submerge beans in water overnight before cooking them. The beans swell with water and cook in much less time. However, soaked beans tend to break up more than unsoaked ones, so it can be beneficial to cook beans from a dry state.

Vegan Chili

If you prefer a meaty chili, you can add some ground beef or ground turkey to this recipe by cooking the beef with the onions. With or without the meat, this hearty chili will keep you full (and satisfied!) for hours.

* Under 500 Calories *

INGREDIENTS | SERVES 8

¼ cup olive oil
2 cups peeled and chopped yellow onion
1 cup peeled and chopped carrots
2 cups chopped and seeded assorted bell peppers
2 teaspoons salt
4 teaspoons ground cumin
1 tablespoon peeled and chopped garlic
2 medium jalapeño peppers, stemmed, seeded, and chopped
1 tablespoon ground ancho chili pepper
1 chipotle in adobo, chopped
1 (28-ounce) can plum tomatoes, roughly chopped, juice included
3 (15.5-ounce) cans beans: 1 red kidney, 1 cannellini, and 1 black, drained and rinsed
1 cup tomato juice
2 tablespoons peeled and finely chopped red onions
2 tablespoons chopped fresh cilantro

1. Heat oil in a large, heavy-bottomed Dutch oven or soup pot over medium heat 1 minute. Add onions, carrots, bell peppers, and salt; cook 15 minutes over medium heat, until onions are soft.
2. In a small dry skillet over medium heat, toast cumin 1 minute. Add garlic, jalapeños, ancho, and chipotle to Dutch oven; cook an additional 5 minutes.
3. Stir in tomatoes, beans, and tomato juice. Simmer covered 45 minutes over low heat.
4. Serve garnished with red onions and cilantro.

Per Serving: | Calories: 263 | Fat: 7.5g | Protein: 10.7g | Sodium: 1,188mg | Fiber: 12.6g | Carbohydrates: 41.0g | Net Carbohydrates: 28.4g | Sugar: 11.4g

Zucchini "Lasagna"

Layered and baked like the beloved Italian-American pasta dish, this wheat-free casserole is best made a day in advance. If you don't have a mandolin or slicing machine, the deli-counter person at your store might be glad to slice your zucchini.

* Under 500 Calories *

INGREDIENTS | SERVES 8

3 cups tomato sauce, divided
4 large zucchini, sliced lengthwise about ⅛" thick, divided
¼ teaspoon salt
¼ teaspoon freshly ground black pepper
1 pound ricotta cheese, divided
1 pound shredded mozzarella cheese, divided
2 cups frozen mixed vegetables, thawed, divided

1. Preheat oven to 350°F.
2. Spread 1 cup tomato sauce onto the bottom of a 9" × 13" baking dish. Arrange a layer of zucchini slices in the pan, slightly overlapping slices.
3. Dot zucchini layer with half of ricotta, distributing teaspoonfuls evenly around casserole. Layer a third of shredded cheese on top of ricotta, then layer half of thawed vegetables.
4. Arrange another layer of zucchini, and repeat fillings, using remaining ricotta, remaining vegetables, and another third shredded cheese. Add final layer of zucchini and spread remaining tomato sauce on top.
5. Sprinkle top with remaining cheese; bake 1 hour until casserole is bubbly and cheese is lightly browned. Cool slightly, about 10 minutes, before cutting and serving.

Per Serving: | Calories: 341 | Fat: 19.2g | Protein: 23.1g | Sodium: 939mg | Fiber: 4.3g | Carbohydrates: 17.4g | Net Carbohydrates: 13.1g | Sugar: 8.1g

Zucchini Lasagna Twist

Try replacing half the zucchini in this recipe with an equal portion of eggplant. Be sure to use thin, flat slices that are very lightly dusted on one side with salt.

Not Your Grandmother's Eggplant Parmigiana

This eggplant parmigiana has all the flavor of your grandmother's recipe but with a healthier twist. The coconut flour and almond meal give the eggplant a nice breading while making this recipe gluten-free.

INGREDIENTS | SERVES 4

¼ cup olive oil, divided

3 large eggs, beaten

½ cup water

1 cup coconut flour

3 cups almond meal

1 medium eggplant (about 1 pound), thinly sliced

1 (24-ounce) jar no-sugar-added tomato sauce, divided

1 pound shredded part-skim mozzarella cheese, divided

1 teaspoon chopped fresh flat-leaf parsley

1. Heat 2 tablespoons oil in a heavy medium skillet over medium heat 1 minute.
2. In small bowl, mix eggs with water. In a second small bowl, add flour. In a third medium bowl, add almond meal.
3. Dip both sides of one eggplant slice in flour and shake off excess; dip coated eggplant slice in egg mixture and shake off excess, then dip both sides of slice into almond meal and shake off excess. Set aside. Repeat process with remaining eggplant slices, adding remaining oil as needed.
4. Fry slices in hot skillet over medium-high heat until golden, about 3 minutes per slice. Drain fried eggplant on a rack or paper towels.
5. Preheat oven to 350°F.
6. Line eggplant slices in a 9" × 13" baking dish. Top each slice with 1 tablespoon tomato sauce, and 1 small mound shredded cheese. Bake until cheese is melted, browning and bubbly, about 15 minutes.
7. Serve garnished with chopped parsley, with remaining tomato sauce on the side.

Per Serving: | Calories: 680 | Fat: 41.9g | Protein: 42.5g | Sodium: 1,672mg | Fiber: 16.3g | Carbohydrates: 34.7g | Net Carbohydrates: 18.4g | Sugar: 14.1g

Chicken Lettuce Cups

These Chicken Lettuce Cups make a great light meal that is also easy to whip up and easy to eat. You can enjoy these cups on their own or pair them with a side of brown rice, if you're incorporating grains into your fasting regimen.

* Under 500 Calories *

INGREDIENTS | SERVES 8

3 pounds ground chicken
⅛ teaspoon finely chopped fresh gingerroot
2 (8-ounce) cans water chestnuts, drained and chopped
¼ cup chili powder
2 tablespoons coconut oil
½ cup coconut aminos
2 tablespoons rice wine vinegar
½ cup chopped scallions, green parts only
1 tablespoon freshly squeezed lime juice
16 large inner leaves of iceberg lettuce, trimmed and chilled

1. In a large bowl, add chicken, ginger, water chestnuts, and chili powder. Combine well with hands.
2. In a large skillet, heat oil on medium heat 1 minute. Add chicken mixture. Use a spatula to cut up chicken into small chunks. Add aminos, vinegar, scallions, and lime juice; cook 8 minutes until chicken is cooked through.
3. Arrange lettuce leaves on a plate and fill each leaf with ¼ cup chicken mixture. Wrap lettuce around mixture. Serve immediately.

Per Serving: | Calories: 305 | Fat: 15.8g | Protein: 29.0g | Sodium: 549mg | Fiber: 2.8g | Carbohydrates: 10.8g | Net Carbohydrates: 8.0g | Sugar: 1.9g

Slow Cooker Chicken Tagine

Tagine is a stew that originated in Morocco and is also found in other areas of North Africa. It's also known as tavas in Cypriot cuisine. Enjoy this easier version of a more traditional tagine recipe!

* Under 500 Calories *

INGREDIENTS | SERVES 4

1½ tablespoons sweet paprika
1 teaspoon ground cinnamon
1½ tablespoons ground coriander
1½ teaspoons ground turmeric
2 teaspoons ground cardamom
1½ teaspoons ground allspice
⅛ teaspoon wheat-free asafetida powder
¼ teaspoon sea salt
¼ teaspoon freshly ground black pepper
4 (5-ounce) skinless, boneless chicken thighs, halved
1 tablespoon olive oil
1½ teaspoons ground ginger
1½ teaspoons saffron
1 (14-ounce) can whole tomatoes, drained
⅓ cup canned chickpeas, thoroughly drained and rinsed
1 quart chicken stock
1 lemon, chopped into wedges
1 tablespoon chopped fresh flat-leaf parsley

1. In a small skillet, toast paprika, cinnamon, coriander, turmeric, cardamom, and allspice until fragrant, about 2 minutes. Set aside and allow to cool 3 minutes.
2. Once cooled, sprinkle spice mixture, asafetida, salt, and pepper on both sides of each half thigh chicken.
3. In a large skillet, heat oil over medium heat 1 minute. Add chicken thighs and sear until browned, about 2 minutes on each side. Remove from heat and place chicken in a 4–6-quart slow cooker.
4. Add ginger to skillet. Cook and stir 2 minutes.
5. Add ginger, saffron, tomatoes, chickpeas, and chicken stock to slow cooker. Cook on high 4 hours. Once done, remove to serving dish and garnish with lemon and parsley.

Per Serving: | Calories: 381 | Fat: 15.8g | Protein: 34.2g | Sodium: 810mg | Fiber: 3.8g | Carbohydrates: 21.5g | Net Carbohydrates: 17.7g | Sugar: 9.4g

Fish Curry

The salmon in this Fish Curry provides a healthy dose of omega-3 fatty acids that can help you fight inflammation and keep your brain healthy.

INGREDIENTS | SERVES 2

1 medium carrot, peeled and chopped
2 cups chicken broth
¼ teaspoon gluten-free fish sauce
1 (13.5-ounce) can unsweetened full-fat coconut milk, refrigerated overnight, cream only
1 medium Roma or vine-ripe tomato, diced
½ small stalk celery, diced
1 tablespoon curry powder
¼ teaspoon ground cumin
¼ teaspoon ground coriander
½ teaspoon ground turmeric
¼ teaspoon freshly grated ginger
2 tablespoons roughly chopped fresh cilantro
½ pound wild-caught salmon, skin removed

1. Boil carrots in a medium saucepan over high heat until softened just slightly, about 3 minutes. Drain, discarding water, and add chicken broth and fish sauce to pan.
2. Add coconut cream, tomato, celery, curry powder, cumin, coriander, and turmeric to pan.
3. Bring to a boil over high heat; cover, reduce heat to low, and simmer 20 minutes, stirring every 5 minutes.
4. Stir in ginger and cilantro. Add fish and stir to cover with liquid.
5. Cook 5 minutes over medium heat to achieve flaky fish, then serve.

Per Serving: | Calories: 592 | Fat: 45.5g | Protein: 29.7g | Sodium: 1,086mg | Fiber: 3.8g | Carbohydrates: 15.2g | Net Carbohydrates: 11.4g | Sugar: 5.1g

Filet Mignon Salad

Filet mignon, the most tender and popular cut of beef, is dressed to the nines in greens, tomatoes, and goat cheese in this filling salad.

INGREDIENTS | SERVES 2

¼ large head romaine lettuce, chopped and ribs removed
½ large head Belgian endive (about 1½ cups), trimmed and thinly sliced crosswise
¼ cup chopped fresh basil
1½ cups baby arugula
2 teaspoons pure maple syrup
½ cup rice wine vinegar
1½ tablespoons freshly squeezed lemon juice
½ teaspoon sea salt
½ teaspoon freshly ground black pepper
½ cup plus 1½ teaspoons olive oil, divided
1 tablespoon unsalted grass-fed butter
½ pound filet mignon
2 ounces crumbled goat cheese
8 cherry tomatoes, halved

1. In a large salad bowl combine romaine, endive, basil, and arugula.
2. In a food processor or blender, add maple syrup, vinegar, lemon juice, salt, and pepper. With machine running on low speed, slowly blend in ½ cup oil. Set aside.
3. Melt butter with remaining olive oil in a medium cast-iron skillet or stainless-steel skillet over medium heat 1 minute. Add filet mignon and cook 7 minutes on each side for medium-rare (or longer, depending on desired degree of doneness). Remove from heat and allow to stand 5 minutes. Slice into strips of medium thickness.
4. Add filet mignon, goat cheese, and cherry tomatoes to salad bowl. Pour in dressing. Toss well to coat, then serve.

Per Serving: | Calories: 910 | Fat: 77.1g | Protein: 36.6g | Sodium: 602mg | Fiber: 4.1g | Carbohydrates: 12.7g | Net Carbohydrates: 8.6g | Sugar: 7.5g

Zoodles with Pesto

Making "zoodles," or zucchini noodles, is not only fun, but is also a healthy way to enjoy pasta recipes.

* Under 500 Calories *

INGREDIENTS | SERVES 3

¾ cup fresh basil leaves
2 tablespoons garlic-infused olive oil
¼ cup pine nuts
2 tablespoons extra-virgin olive oil
½ cup freshly grated Parmesan cheese
¼ teaspoon sea salt, divided
¼ teaspoon freshly ground black pepper, divided
1 tablespoon olive oil
1 pound zucchini, peeled into long, narrow ribbons

1. For pesto sauce, combine basil, garlic oil, and pine nuts in a food processor and pulse until coarsely chopped. Add olive oil, cheese, ⅛ teaspoon salt, and ⅛ teaspoon pepper and process until smooth.

2. Heat olive oil in a medium sauté pan over medium heat 1 minute. Add zucchini noodles, ⅛ teaspoon salt, and ⅛ teaspoon pepper to pan and stir 5 minutes until noodles are tender. Serve with pesto sauce.

Per Serving: | Calories: 374 | Fat: 32.8g | Protein: 8.9g | Sodium: 443mg | Fiber: 2.3g | Carbohydrates: 9.1g | Net Carbohydrates: 6.8g | Sugar: 4.1g

Flavored Oils

To infuse oil with flavor and complexity, stuff herbs, spices, and garlic cloves into a bottle of the oil and steep for at least three days—up to two weeks. Fine olive oil becomes a transcendent condiment when perfumed by rosemary, thyme, savory, garlic, peppercorns, dried mushrooms, or truffles. You can also buy infused oils at gourmet stores.

Chicken Burgers

This basic recipe will become a staple for your intermittent fasting regimen. Chicken Burgers are easy to whip up and they store well, so you can always have a quick meal on the go. You can also make them your own by substituting any type of meat and spices.

* Under 500 Calories *

INGREDIENTS | SERVES 4

1 pound ground chicken
½ teaspoon salt
½ teaspoon ground white pepper
1 large egg, beaten
¼ cup grated Parmesan cheese
1 tablespoon olive oil

1. In a large bowl, mix all ingredients except oil together with your hands until well blended.
2. Shape mixture into 4 patties.
3. In a large skillet heat oil on medium-high 1 minute and add burgers. Brown on one side about 5 minutes, then flip and cook other side, another 5 minutes until cooked through.

Per Serving: | Calories: 224 | Fat: 13.9g | Protein: 21.9g | Sodium: 480mg | Fiber: 0.9g | Carbohydrates: 1.2g | Net Carbohydrates: 0.3g | Sugar: 0.1g

Pork and Fennel Meatballs

These meatballs can be described as earthy and definitely tasty. Serve either as appetizers or as a full meal with pasta and marinara sauce with a sprinkle of chopped fresh parsley.

* Under 500 Calories *

INGREDIENTS | YIELDS 24 MEATBALLS

1 pound 84 percent lean ground pork
2 tablespoons roughly chopped fresh flat-leaf parsley
3 tablespoons almond meal
1 large egg
¼ teaspoon salt
½ teaspoon freshly ground black pepper
1½ tablespoons olive oil
2 teaspoons fennel seeds

1. In a mixing bowl, combine pork, parsley, almond meal, egg, salt, and pepper. Shape mixture into 24 (1") meatballs.
2. In a medium skillet, heat oil over medium heat 1 minute and sauté fennel seeds until fragrant, about 4 minutes.
3. Add meatballs to pan. Brown meatballs on all sides, about 20 minutes total. Meatballs are cooked through when no longer pink inside.

Per Serving: 1 meatball | Calories: 54 | Fat: 4.1g | Protein: 3.9g | Sodium: 38mg | Fiber: 0.2g | Carbohydrates: 0.3g | Net Carbohydrates: 0.1g | Sugar: 0.0g

Citrus Flank Steak

This citrusy steak pairs perfectly with a garden salad garnished with strawberries or blueberries.

* Under 500 Calories *

INGREDIENTS | SERVES 6

¼ cup toasted sesame oil
1 tablespoon freshly squeezed lime juice
1 tablespoon pineapple juice
1 tablespoon pure maple syrup
1 (5") knob ginger, peeled and thinly sliced
¼ teaspoon salt
¼ teaspoon freshly ground black pepper
1 (1½-pound) flank steak
2 teaspoons olive oil

1. In a food processor, mix sesame oil, lime juice, pineapple juice, maple syrup, ginger, salt, and pepper until smooth; pour into a large bowl.
2. Add steak to bowl and cover with marinade. Refrigerate covered 4 hours.
3. Heat olive oil in a large cast-iron skillet over medium heat 1 minute, or heat grill to medium-high.
4. Cook steak in skillet or grill steak 8 minutes on each side. Transfer steak to a cutting board; cover loosely with foil and let rest 10 minutes.
5. Slice steak against the grain and serve.

Per Serving: | Calories: 333 | Fat: 27.5g | Protein: 16.3g | Sodium: 52mg | Fiber: 0.0g | Carbohydrates: 0.3g | Net Carbohydrates: 0.3g | Sugar: 0.2g

Stuffed Peppers with Ground Turkey

These stuffed peppers store very well, so you can make them in advance. This recipe is also a basic template, so feel free to add any extra vegetables that you have on hand.

INGREDIENTS | SERVES 3

1 tablespoon olive oil
1 pound ground turkey
1 tablespoon garlic-infused oil, divided
2 medium Roma tomatoes, chopped
2 tablespoons pine nuts
1 cup cooked brown rice
1½ teaspoons chili powder
½ teaspoon ground cumin
1 teaspoon smoked paprika
3 tablespoons chopped fresh cilantro
3 large bell peppers (1 orange, 1 yellow, 1 green), stemmed, halved, and seeded
2 tablespoons coconut oil, melted
6 (1-ounce) slices goat cheese
3 tablespoons no-sugar-added salsa

1. Preheat oven to 375°F.
2. Heat olive oil in a large skillet over medium-high heat 1 minute. Add turkey and cook until browned, about 7 minutes.
3. Add half of garlic oil to skillet along with tomatoes and pine nuts; stir and heat through, about 3 minutes.
4. Add brown rice and stir to combine. Stir in remaining half of garlic oil as well as chili powder, cumin, paprika, and cilantro. Remove from heat.
5. Stuff halved peppers with brown rice mixture and brush outside of peppers with coconut oil. Place peppers in an 9" × 13" shallow baking dish. Top each pepper with a slice of goat cheese. Loosely cover dish with foil.
6. Bake 40 minutes until peppers are tender. Garnish with salsa and serve.

Per Serving: | Calories: 779 | Fat: 49.4g | Protein: 43.6g | Sodium: 487mg | Fiber: 5.7g | Carbohydrates: 31.0g | Net Carbohydrates: 25.3g | Sugar: 6.7g

Beef with Spinach and Sweet Potatoes

This Beef with Spinach and Sweet Potatoes is a perfectly complete meal all in one. You'll enjoy a great balance of high-quality protein, vegetables, and carbohydrates.

INGREDIENTS | SERVES 4

1 pound organic or grass-fed beef tenderloin, cut into 4 medallions

¼ teaspoon salt

¼ teaspoon freshly ground black pepper

3 teaspoons olive oil, divided

½ pound sweet potatoes, peeled and cut into ½" cubes

½ teaspoon ground turmeric

¼ teaspoon chili powder

2 tablespoons rice wine vinegar

3 tablespoons pure maple syrup

1½ cups fresh baby spinach

⅓ cup toasted pumpkin seeds

1. Season beef with salt and pepper. Heat 2 teaspoons oil in a 9" cast-iron skillet over medium-high heat 1 minute. Add beef to skillet and cook 3 minutes on both sides for medium-rare. Transfer to plate and cover with foil.
2. Add remaining oil to skillet along with sweet potatoes. Cook over medium-high heat until browned, about 15 minutes. Stir in turmeric and chili powder and cook an additional 1 minute.
3. Add vinegar and maple syrup to skillet. If potatoes start to stick, add more vinegar. Add spinach, ½ cup at a time, and cook 2 minutes, stirring.
4. Transfer spinach and sweet potatoes to plates and top with beef, followed by equal amounts of pumpkin seeds on each.

Per Serving: | Calories: 779 | Fat: 49.4g | Protein: 43.6g | Sodium: 487mg | Fiber: 5.7g | Carbohydrates: 31.0g | Net Carbohydrates: 25.3g | Sugar: 6.7g

Lemon Thyme Chicken

Lemon and thyme pair together to make this delicious citrus chicken—but it's not just flavor that thyme offers. This herb has also been shown to help lower blood pressure and cholesterol levels and may even improve your mood.

* Under 500 Calories *

INGREDIENTS | SERVES 4

4 chicken thighs and 4 chicken drumsticks (approximately ½ pound of each)

3 medium lemons, halved

Zest of 1 medium lemon

1 tablespoon unsalted grass-fed butter, melted

¼ teaspoon sea salt

½ teaspoon freshly ground black pepper

2 tablespoons fresh thyme leaves

6 fresh basil leaves, torn

1. Preheat oven to 375°F.
2. In a large bowl, add chicken. Squeeze juice from lemons into bowl.
3. Add lemon zest, butter, salt, pepper, and thyme; toss well with your hands. Place chicken in a 9" × 13" baking dish.
4. Bake chicken 40 minutes, basting every 10 minutes. Skin should get crispy and meat should be cooked through.
5. Garnish with basil leaves and serve.

Per Serving: | Calories: 480 | Fat: 22.5g | Protein: 58.6g | Sodium: 380mg | Fiber: 0.5g | Carbohydrates: 2.3g | Net Carbohydrates: 1.8g | Sugar: 0.6g

Spinach and Feta–Stuffed Chicken Breasts

This recipe is easy to make and only requires a few ingredients. You'll be just 30 minutes away from a delicious meal when it's time to break your fast.

* Under 500 Calories *

INGREDIENTS | SERVES 2

1 tablespoon garlic-infused olive oil
1 cup fresh spinach leaves
½ cup crumbled feta cheese
2 (4-ounce) boneless, skinless chicken breasts, pounded to ¼" thickness
1 large egg, lightly beaten
1 cup almond meal

1. Preheat oven to 350°F.
2. Heat oil in a medium skillet over low heat 1 minute. Cook spinach until soft, about 3 minutes. Add feta, stir a few times, and remove from heat.
3. Place half of spinach mixture on each chicken breast. Wrap chicken around mixture and secure with toothpicks.
4. In a shallow bowl, add egg. In a separate shallow bowl, add almond meal. Roll each breast in egg, tap off any excess, then roll in almond meal until well coated.
5. Place chicken in an 8" × 8" casserole dish. Bake 30 minutes and serve.

Per Serving: | Calories: 395 | Fat: 24.1g | Protein: 35.8g | Sodium: 423mg | Fiber: 1.8g | Carbohydrates: 5.2g | Net Carbohydrates: 3.4g | Sugar: 2.1g

Easy Pan Chicken

This makes for a comforting home-cooked meal that's easy to assemble and ready in less than 45 minutes.

INGREDIENTS | SERVES 4

3 tablespoons whole-grain mustard
2 teaspoons dried oregano
1 teaspoon dried thyme
1 tablespoon unsalted grass-fed butter, softened
2 teaspoons Dijon mustard
4 bone-in chicken thighs and 4 drumsticks (about 2 pounds), patted dry
½ teaspoon salt
1 teaspoon freshly ground black pepper
⅔ cup almond meal
4 medium carrots, peeled and halved lengthwise
1 tablespoon garlic-infused olive oil

1. Preheat oven to 425°F.
2. In a small bowl, combine whole-grain mustard, oregano, thyme, butter, and Dijon mustard.
3. Season chicken with salt and pepper. Rub mustard-butter mixture all over chicken.
4. In a wide bowl, add almond meal. Dip chicken in meal, coating evenly.
5. Place carrots cut side down with chicken on an ungreased baking sheet and drizzle with olive oil.
6. Bake until chicken is golden and no longer pink, about 40 minutes. Serve warm.

Per Serving: | Calories: 663 | Fat: 36.4g | Protein: 62.9g | Sodium: 914mg | Fiber: 4.2g | Carbohydrates: 13.3g | Net Carbohydrates: 9.1g | Sugar: 3.6g

Pumpkin Maple Roast Chicken

Once in the oven, this simple roast chicken with pumpkin, maple syrup, cinnamon, and thyme will cast a fragrant spell over your kitchen.

INGREDIENTS | SERVES 4

1½ tablespoons unsalted grass-fed butter
1 tablespoon canned pumpkin
1 tablespoon pure maple syrup
1 teaspoon ground cinnamon
1 teaspoon dried thyme
½ teaspoon sea salt
¼ teaspoon freshly ground black pepper
1 (4-pound) whole chicken

1. Preheat oven to 375°F.
2. Melt butter in a small saucepan over medium-high heat 1 minute. Stir in pumpkin, maple syrup, cinnamon, thyme, salt, and pepper. Refrigerate 10 minutes.
3. Cut small slit under skin on both sides of chicken breasts and behind legs. Once the pumpkin mixture is cool, generously rub it under skin and all over top of skin. Place chicken breast side up on the rack of a large roasting pan. Roast 60 minutes until a meat thermometer registers 165°F at thickest part of thigh.
4. Tent chicken with foil and let rest 5 minutes before carving.

Per Serving: | Calories: 526 | Fat: 29.9g | Protein: 50.4g | Sodium: 361mg | Fiber: 0.6g | Carbohydrates: 4.4g | Net Carbohydrates: 3.8g | Sugar: 3.2g

Canned Pumpkin

There is a very similar-looking canned product known as pumpkin pie filling. Pumpkin pie filling contains less healthy ingredients such as sugar, high-fructose corn syrup, and artificial flavorings and colorings. Pure canned pumpkin should be nothing but pumpkin.

Salmon with Herbs

Salmon is one of the best fatty fish to consume because it's rich in omega-3 fatty acids and doesn't contain a lot of mercury like bigger fish do. However, you can tweak this recipe and use any fish that you like.

*** Under 500 Calories ***

INGREDIENTS | SERVES 4

1 (1-pound) salmon fillet
¼ teaspoon salt
½ teaspoon freshly ground black pepper
¼ cup plus 2 tablespoons olive oil
¼ cup chopped fresh dill
2 tablespoons roughly chopped fresh rosemary
¼ cup fresh flat-leaf parsley
2 tablespoons fresh thyme leaves
2 tablespoons freshly squeezed lemon juice

1. Preheat oven to 250°F.
2. Coat a 9" × 13" baking dish with cooking spray. Lay salmon skin side down and sprinkle with salt and pepper.
3. Blend olive oil with dill, rosemary, parsley, thyme, and lemon juice in a small food processor. Use a spatula or your hands to pat herb paste over salmon.
4. Bake salmon 22–28 minutes depending on thickness. Insert tines of a fork into thickest part of fillet and gently pull. If fish flakes easily, it is done.
5. Slide a spatula under fish and set on a cutting board. Cut into equal pieces and serve.

Per Serving: | Calories: 342 | Fat: 26.2g | Protein: 22.8g | Sodium: 197mg | Fiber: 0.5g | Carbohydrates: 1.5g | Net Carbohydrates: 1.0g | Sugar: 0.2g

Mediterranean Flaky Fish with Vegetables

The lovely flavors of the Mediterranean are paired with flaky fish in this recipe, creating a healthy and tasty dinner. Pair with a salad and potatoes.

* Under 500 Calories *

INGREDIENTS | SERVES 4

4 (3.5-ounce) skinless Atlantic cod fillets
1 cup grated zucchini
¼ cup thinly sliced fresh basil, plus 4 whole basil leaves, divided
20 cherry tomatoes, halved
10 black olives, sliced
¼ teaspoon salt
½ teaspoon freshly ground black pepper
4 tablespoons dry white wine, divided
4 tablespoons olive oil, divided

1. Preheat oven to 400°F.
2. To make parchment pockets: cut a 17" × 11" piece of parchment paper. With one longer edge closest to you, fold in half from left to right. Using scissors, cut out a large heart shape, using the fold as the center of the heart and cutting half of a heart shape. Repeat to cut four hearts in all. On a large cutting board, lay down one parchment heart and place fish on half of heart, leaving at least a 1½" border around fillet. Repeat with remaining fish fillets. Lay parchment hearts in a 9" × 13" baking dish.
3. In a medium bowl, combine zucchini, sliced basil, tomatoes, olives, salt, and pepper. Stir to combine.
4. Evenly distribute vegetable mixture over each fish fillet in parchment hearts.
5. Take the free side of each parchment heart and fold over fish, making both edges of the heart line up. Starting at rounded end, crimp and fold edges together tightly. Leave a few inches at pointed end unfolded. Grab pointed edge and tilt heart to pour in 1 tablespoon each of wine and oil. Repeat for each heart. Finish by crimping edges and twisting pointed ends around and under pockets.
6. Bake fish until just cooked through, about 12 minutes. Poke a toothpick through parchment paper. Fish should be done if toothpick easily slides through fish. Carefully cut open packets (steam will escape). Garnish with whole basil leaves and serve.

Per Serving: | Calories: 230 | Fat: 14.8g | Protein: 16.5g | Sodium: 533mg | Fiber: 1.8g | Carbohydrates: 5.5g | Net Carbohydrates: 3.7g | Sugar: 3.1g

What Are Other Fish Options?

Other great options for this recipe are striped bass and halibut. These white fish have a mild taste that is similar to cod and won't affect the flavor profile of this recipe.

Basic Baked Scallops

This yummy seafood recipe takes less than 30 minutes to make and pairs well with green beans or a side salad.

INGREDIENTS | SERVES 2

¾ pound sea scallops
2 tablespoons freshly squeezed lemon juice
2½ tablespoons unsalted grass-fed butter, melted
¼ teaspoon sea salt
½ teaspoon freshly ground black pepper
2 tablespoons chopped fresh flat-leaf parsley
½ cup almond meal
½ teaspoon smoked paprika
2 tablespoons olive oil

1. Preheat oven to 425°F.
2. Toss together scallops, lemon juice, melted butter, salt, and pepper in a 2-quart baking dish.
3. In a medium bowl, combine parsley, almond meal, paprika, and olive oil. Sprinkle mixture on top of scallops.
4. Bake scallops 14 minutes until they are heated through and almond meal is golden. Serve immediately.

Per Serving: | Calories: 540 | Fat: 42.7g | Protein: 26.8g | Sodium: 907mg | Fiber: 3.5g | Carbohydrates: 13.4g | Net Carbohydrates: 9.9g | Sugar: 1.5g

Mushroom Pork Medallions

These Mushroom Pork Medallions are gluten-free, Paleo-approved, and extremely delicious. The flax meal adds a rich, nutty flavor as well as omega-3 fatty acids and antioxidants.

* Under 500 Calories *

INGREDIENTS | SERVES 2

1 tablespoon olive oil
1 pound pork tenderloin, sliced into ½"-thick medallions
1 small yellow onion, peeled and sliced
¼ cup sliced white mushrooms
1 clove garlic, peeled and minced
2 teaspoons flax meal
½ cup no-salt-added beef broth
¼ teaspoon dried rosemary, crushed
⅛ teaspoon freshly ground black pepper

1. In a large skillet, heat olive oil over medium-high heat 30 seconds. Add pork and brown 2 minutes on each side. Remove pork from skillet and set aside.
2. In same skillet, add onion, mushrooms, and garlic and sauté 1 minute. Stir in flax meal until blended.
3. Gradually stir in broth, rosemary, and pepper. Bring to a boil over high heat. Cook and stir 1 minute until thickened.
4. Lay pork medallions over mixture in skillet. Reduce heat to low; cover and simmer 15 minutes until meat juices run clear.

Per Serving: | Calories: 311 | Fat: 13.2g | Protein: 40.7g | Sodium: 433mg | Fiber: 1.3g | Carbohydrates: 5.8g | Net Carbohydrates: 4.5g | Sugar: 2.1g

Slow Cooker Mediterranean Stew

The Mediterranean region is an excellent climate for growing many foods and spices with a high nutrient content. This stew uses slow-cooking methods to extract as many of those nutrients as possible.

* Under 500 Calories *

INGREDIENTS | SERVES 8

1 medium butternut squash, peeled, seeded, and cubed
2 cups cubed eggplant, with peel
2 cups cubed zucchini
1 (10-ounce) package frozen okra, thawed
1 cup puréed fresh tomatoes
1 cup peeled and chopped yellow onion
1 large vine-ripened tomato, chopped
1 medium carrot, peeled and thinly sliced
½ cup vegetable broth
1 clove garlic, peeled
½ teaspoon ground cumin
½ teaspoon ground turmeric
¼ teaspoon crushed red pepper flakes
¼ teaspoon ground cinnamon
¼ teaspoon paprika

Combine all ingredients in a 4–6-quart slow cooker and cook on low 10 hours. Serve warm.

Per Serving: | Calories: 82 | Fat: 0.3g | Protein: 3.0g | Sodium: 56mg | Fiber: 4.7g | Carbohydrates: 19.6g | Net Carbohydrates: 14.9g | Sugar: 7.5g

Mediterranean Lamb Stew

Start by seasoning 1 pound of cubed lamb with salt and pepper. Heat a large sauté pan over medium heat 30 seconds and add olive oil. When the oil is hot, add the lamb. Sauté until each side is brown, about 1 minute per side. Add the lamb to your slow cooker with the other ingredients and cook 10 hours.

Mexican-Style Chili

The flavors in this Mexican-Style Chili develop even more as it sits in the refrigerator, so don't be afraid to make it in advance. You can even freeze some of it for later and store it for up to 3 months.

* Under 500 Calories *

INGREDIENTS | SERVES 10

2 tablespoons olive oil

5 pounds boneless beef chuck stew meat, cut into 1" pieces

2 teaspoons salt

½ teaspoon freshly ground black pepper

¾ cup chicken broth

2 green chilies, seeded and diced

3 tablespoons Mexican-style chili powder

3 celery stalks, chopped

4 cloves garlic, peeled and minced

1 medium yellow onion, peeled and chopped

2 large beefsteak tomatoes, diced

1. In a large skillet, add oil and beef and cook over medium heat 10 minutes until brown on the outside. Season with salt and pepper.
2. In a 4–6-quart slow cooker, add broth, chilies, chili powder, celery, garlic, onions, tomatoes, and cooked beef. Cook on high 4 hours. Serve warm.

Per Serving: | Calories: 401 | Fat: 15.5g | Protein: 60.2g | Sodium: 733mg | Fiber: 1.8g | Carbohydrates: 5.4g | Net Carbohydrates: 3.6g | Sugar: 2.3g

Pepper Steak

You can combine this zesty steak with a simple garden salad for a complete, balanced meal that's easy to prepare and full of nutrients.

INGREDIENTS | SERVES 2

2 (6-ounce) New York sirloins, sliced into thin strips

1 cup coconut aminos

4 garlic cloves, peeled and chopped

1 (1") knob ginger, peeled and sliced

2 medium shallots, diced

10 mini sweet peppers, seeded and sliced

2 teaspoons freshly cracked black peppercorns

½ teaspoon sea salt

2 tablespoons olive oil

2 cups cooked brown rice

1. Marinate steak strips in coconut aminos 20 minutes.
2. In a large sauté pan over medium heat, cook garlic, ginger, shallots, sweet peppers, and seasonings with olive oil 5 minutes.
3. Add steak strips to the pan and cook 3 minutes. Flip strips and cook an additional 3 minutes.
4. Remove steak strips and peppers from heat and drain off excess oils. Serve ingredients over bed of brown rice.

Per Serving: | Calories: 847 | Fat: 36.2g | Protein: 44.2g | Sodium: 747mg | Fiber: 11.1g | Carbohydrates: 73.2g | Net Carbohydrates: 61.1g | Sugar: 14.2g

Sirloin Steak Fact

The New York loin (or New York strip), which is also known as strip loin and Kansas City strip steak, is taken from the short loin of the cow. The muscle that makes up this steak does very little work and therefore is a tender cut of meat.

CHAPTER 10

Snacks

Artichoke Dip

This Artichoke Dip is a lighter version of the original with all of the same delicious flavor. You can serve it alongside your favorite vegetables or gluten-free crackers.

INGREDIENTS | SERVES 8

2 (14-ounce) cans quartered artichoke hearts, drained, rinsed, and chopped

1 medium red bell pepper, stemmed, seeded, and finely chopped

1 medium green bell pepper, stemmed, seeded, and finely chopped

3 cloves garlic, peeled and minced

2 cups homemade mayonnaise

¼ teaspoon ground white pepper

1 pound grated Parmesan cheese, divided

1. Preheat oven to 325°F.
2. Mix all ingredients except ¼ pound Parmesan cheese. Spread mixture into a 9" × 9" baking dish and sprinkle remaining Parmesan on top.
3. Bake 45 minutes until golden brown.

Per Serving: | Calories: 643 | Fat: 53.9g | Protein: 17.8g | Sodium: 1,616mg | Fiber: 2.1g | Carbohydrates: 14.0g | Net Carbohydrates: 11.9g

Curry Dip

The jalapeños in this dip give it a little bit of a kick, but if you prefer it less spicy, you can omit the jalapeños altogether, or use finely diced green peppers in their place.

*** Under 500 Calories ***

INGREDIENTS | YIELDS 2½ CUPS

1 teaspoon olive oil
½ cup peeled and finely chopped yellow onion
½ medium jalapeño pepper, stemmed, seeded, and finely chopped (about 1 teaspoon)
2 teaspoons seeded and finely chopped red bell pepper
1 teaspoon curry powder
1 teaspoon ground cumin
½ teaspoon ground coriander
½ teaspoon ground turmeric
⅛ teaspoon cayenne pepper
¼ teaspoon salt
1 tablespoon soft raisins
1 tablespoon water
1½ cups mayonnaise
1 tablespoon chopped fresh cilantro
⅛ teaspoon freshly squeezed lemon juice

1. Heat oil 30 seconds in a small skillet over medium heat. Add onion, jalapeño, and red pepper; cook 5 minutes, stirring occasionally until onions are translucent. Add curry powder, cumin, coriander, turmeric, cayenne, and salt. Cook an additional minute until spices are very fragrant. Add raisins and water.
2. Transfer mixture to a food processor. Chop on high speed 30 seconds. Scrape down sides of bowl with a rubber spatula. Add mayonnaise and cilantro; process an additional 30 seconds until smooth and even. Add lemon juice and serve.

Per Serving: ½ cup | Calories: 174 | Fat: 17.2g | Protein: 0.7g | Sodium: 257mg | Fiber: 0.8g | Carbohydrates: 4.2g | Net Carbohydrates: 3.4g | Sugar: 2.2g

What Is "Curry Powder"?

What we know as "curry powder" is actually a blend of spices, invented by the British to resemble one of the famous masalas (spice blends) of India. Most authentic Indian recipes call not for curry powder but a combination of spices (a masala) specifically designed for that dish.

Salsa Fresca (Pico de Gallo)

This basic Salsa Fresca is the perfect addition to any fish or chicken dish. You can also eat it with gluten-free crackers for a quick snack.

* Under 500 Calories *

INGREDIENTS | SERVES 8

4 medium vine-ripened tomatoes, seeded and finely diced, divided
1 small white onion, peeled and finely chopped
1 medium jalapeño pepper, stemmed, seeded, and finely chopped
1 tablespoon puréed chipotle in adobo
½ teaspoon salt
2 teaspoons freshly squeezed lime juice
¼ cup chopped fresh cilantro

1. In a blender or food processor, purée a third of tomatoes. Combine in a medium bowl with remaining tomato, onion, jalapeño, chipotle purée, salt, lime juice, and cilantro.
2. Serve. Best if used within 2 days.

Per Serving: | Calories: 15 | Fat: 0.1g | Protein: 0.7g | Sodium: 148mg | Fiber: 1.0g | Carbohydrates: 3.6g | Net Carbohydrates: 2.6g | Sugar: 2.2g

Roasted Beets

Roasting brings natural juices to the surface of these magenta roots and caramelizes them into a sweet, intensely flavored crust. Snacking on beets can curb sugar cravings so you're less likely to indulge in unhealthy foods during your feeding window.

* Under 500 Calories *

INGREDIENTS | SERVES 8

2 pounds (about 8 large) beets, cut into 1" wedges
1 tablespoon olive oil
¼ teaspoon ground cinnamon
¼ teaspoon salt
¼ teaspoon chopped fresh flat-leaf parsley

1. Preheat oven to 350°F.
2. Toss beets with olive oil, cinnamon, and salt. Spread into a single layer on a nonstick baking sheet.
3. Roast on the middle rack of oven until tender, about 1 hour, turning once after 30 minutes. Serve sprinkled with chopped parsley.

Per Serving: | Calories: 52 | Fat: 1.7g | Protein: 1.4g | Sodium: 139mg | Fiber: 2.5g | Carbohydrates: 8.3g | Net Carbohydrates: 5.8g | Sugar: 5.8g

Cooking Beets—Preserving Nutrition

The flavorful, nutrient-rich juices in beets are water-soluble. To lock in the sweetness, color, and food value of these wonderful vegetables, cook them in their skins. When boiling them, put a few drops of red wine vinegar in the water, which also helps seal in beet juices.

Rutabaga Oven Fries

Though not really fried, these golden batons look and feel like French fries and are great for dipping in ketchup or aioli.

* Under 500 Calories *

INGREDIENTS | SERVES 4

1 large rutabaga ("wax turnip"), thickly peeled and sliced in sticks 2½" × ½"
1 tablespoon olive oil
¼ teaspoon salt
1 tablespoon finely chopped fresh thyme leaves
¼ teaspoon freshly ground black pepper

1. Preheat oven to 400°F.
2. Soak rutabaga sticks, or "batons," in cold water 30 minutes. Dry thoroughly with paper towels. Toss gently with oil and salt.
3. Spread fries in a single layer on an ungreased sheet pan and bake, turning occasionally, until lightly browned and tender, about 30 minutes. Remove from oven and toss with thyme and pepper.

Per Serving: | Calories: 102 | Fat: 3.5g | Protein: 2.2g | Sodium: 168mg | Fiber: 4.6g | Carbohydrates: 17.0g | Net Carbohydrates: 12.4g | Sugar: 8.6g

Mushroom-Stuffed Tomatoes

Use any kind of ripe tomatoes you prefer for this dish. Late in the season, Roma plum tomatoes are usually the best choice, since they keep a long time even when ripe. If using a processor to chop the mushrooms, "pulse" them in small batches, stopping before they clump.

* Under 500 Calories *

INGREDIENTS | SERVES 6

4 medium shallots, peeled and finely chopped
2 tablespoons olive oil, divided
1 pound white mushrooms, finely chopped
1¼ teaspoons salt, divided
¼ cup white wine
¼ cup finely chopped fresh flat-leaf parsley
¼ teaspoon freshly ground black pepper
6 large ripe tomatoes, halved crosswise, rounded ends trimmed flat
3 tablespoons almond meal

1. Preheat oven to 350°F.
2. Sauté chopped shallots with 1 tablespoon olive oil 1 minute in a large skillet over medium heat. Add mushrooms and 1 teaspoon salt, and raise heat to high. Cook, stirring occasionally, about 5 minutes, until mushrooms have given up their water and most water has evaporated.
3. Add white wine to skillet and cook an additional 5 minutes until wine has mostly evaporated. Stir in parsley, remove from heat, and season with black pepper.
4. Scoop innards from tomatoes and season tomato cups with remaining salt. Fill each tomato with mushroom filling so that it mounds slightly, topping each mound with a sprinkle of almond meal.
5. Place stuffed tomatoes in a 9" × 13" baking dish and drizzle with remaining olive oil. Bake 25 minutes until soft.

Per Serving: | Calories: 106 | Fat: 6.4g | Protein: 4.2g | Sodium: 495mg | Fiber: 2.7g | Carbohydrates: 9.3g | Net Carbohydrates: 6.6g | Sugar: 5.1g

Onion Jam

The concentrated sweetness and naturally complex flavor of this caramelized onion spread come from slow cooking, which breaks down the cell walls of the onions, releasing 100 percent of their flavor. Serve it with gluten-free crackers or Paleo Chips (see recipe in this chapter).

*** Under 500 Calories ***

INGREDIENTS | SERVES 8

2 tablespoons olive oil
2 sprigs fresh thyme, stems removed
8 large white onions, peeled, halved, and sliced thinly across the grain
½ teaspoon salt

1. Heat oil in a large, heavy-bottomed Dutch oven over medium heat 1 minute until oil shimmers but does not smoke. Add thyme and sliced onions. Sprinkle with salt.
2. Reduce heat to low; cook slowly, stirring gently with a wooden spoon. As onions begin to caramelize (turn brown), use the wooden spoon to scrape dried-on juices from the bottom of the pot; stir regularly to incorporate as much of these browned juices as possible. Cook this way until onions are dark brown and mostly disintegrated into a thick spread, about 40 minutes total.
3. Remove from heat and cool to room temperature, or serve warm.

Per Serving: | Calories: 89 | Fat: 3.4g | Protein: 1.7g | Sodium: 151mg | Fiber: 2.6g | Carbohydrates: 14.0g | Net Carbohydrates: 11.4g | Sugar: 6.4g

Stuffed Eggs

These filled eggs are a variation on deviled eggs and make a great first course or garnish for a main-course salad. Their tops are attractively browned under the broiler.

* Under 500 Calories *

INGREDIENTS | SERVES 8

8 large hard-boiled eggs, peeled and halved lengthwise
¼ cup Dijon mustard
3 tablespoons unsweetened full-fat coconut milk
2 tablespoons finely chopped shallots
1 tablespoon rice wine vinegar
1 tablespoon chopped fresh chives
1 tablespoon chopped fresh tarragon
¼ teaspoon salt
¼ teaspoon ground white pepper
¼ cup unsalted grass-fed butter

1. Turn on oven broiler to low.
2. Remove egg yolks from whites and combine with mustard, milk, shallots, vinegar, chives, and tarragon. Season with salt and pepper. Transfer mixture to a piping bag and pipe into egg whites (or you can also use a spoon).
3. Place filled eggs in a 9" × 13" baking dish. Dot tops with butter and broil until tops are lightly browned, about 5 minutes. Serve warm.

Per Serving: | Calories: 161 | Fat: 12.3g | Protein: 7.1g | Sodium: 340mg | Fiber: 0.1g | Carbohydrates: 1.9g | Net Carbohydrates: 1.8g | Sugar: 0.8g

Cinnamon Spice Granola

This granola is excellent to have on hand when you need a little snack to hold you over until your next meal. Keep a small container in your car or at work so you always have a healthy option ready to go.

* Under 500 Calories *

INGREDIENTS | SERVES 8

2 cups gluten-free quick-cooking oats
1 cup walnut pieces
1 teaspoon ground cinnamon
½ teaspoon ground nutmeg
¼ teaspoon ground cloves
3 tablespoons coconut sugar
¼ cup pure maple syrup
¼ cup coconut oil, melted

1. Preheat oven to 350°F.
2. In a large bowl, combine all ingredients.
3. Spread mixture in an even layer on an ungreased baking sheet and bake 20 minutes. Stir once halfway through baking.
4. Allow to cool 15 minutes before serving.

Per Serving: | Calories: 387 | Fat: 23.1g | Protein: 7.8g | Sodium: 2mg | Fiber: 5.0g | Carbohydrates: 37.4g | Net Carbohydrates: 32.4g | Sugar: 15.1g

A Note about Oats

If you have digestive troubles, it may be helpful to stick to just ¼ cup of oats at a time. Servings larger than that may bring on uncomfortable symptoms, due to the oats' high fiber content.

Cranberry Almond Granola

This Cranberry Almond Granola makes a delicious snack all on its own, but you can make it a meal by throwing it on top of some coconut-milk yogurt or pouring coconut or almond milk on top and garnishing with sliced banana.

* Under 500 Calories *

INGREDIENTS | YIELDS 2½ CUPS

1 tablespoon whole walnuts
1 tablespoon flaxseeds
1 cup gluten-free rolled oats
1 tablespoon raw slivered almonds
½ teaspoon ground cinnamon
3 tablespoons coconut oil, melted
3 tablespoons pure maple syrup
¼ teaspoon alcohol-free vanilla extract
¼ teaspoon alcohol-free almond extract
2 tablespoons no-sugar-added dried cranberries

1. Preheat oven to 350°F.
2. Using a food processor or blender, pulse walnuts until ground. Transfer to a large bowl. Next add flaxseed to processor and pulse until finely ground. Transfer to large bowl with walnuts. Add oats, almonds, and cinnamon to bowl. Stir to combine.
3. In a medium bowl, stir together oil, maple syrup, vanilla extract, and almond extract. Pour over oat mixture in large bowl and combine.
4. Spread granola on a rimmed, ungreased baking sheet and bake 15 minutes. Stir occasionally to ensure granola turns a light brown color.
5. Remove from oven and add cranberries, stirring to combine. Store in an airtight container up to 3 weeks.

Per Serving: ¼ cup | Calories: 105 | Fat: 5.8g | Protein: 1.9g | Sodium: 1mg | Fiber: 1.6g | Carbohydrates: 11.4g | Net Carbohydrates: 9.8g | Sugar: 4.0g

Choosing Dried Cranberries

When looking for dried cranberries, pay close attention to the ingredients list. Many companies try to counteract the natural tartness of the cranberries by adding sugar or corn syrup. Choose a brand that contains only dried cranberries or dried cranberries that have been sweetened with pure fruit juice.

Mini Baked Eggplant Pizza Bites

These Mini Baked Eggplant Pizza Bites give you all the flavor of pizza with significantly more nutrients—and no gluten. They make a great grab-and-go snack or a mini-meal all on their own.

★ Under 500 Calories ★

INGREDIENTS | SERVES 4

2 medium eggplants, top and bottom ends cut off, cut into round slices, approximately ¼" thick
½ teaspoon salt
1 large egg, whisked
¾ cup almond meal
2 tablespoons dried oregano
2 tablespoons olive oil
½ cup marinara sauce
¼ cup shredded mozzarella cheese

1. Preheat oven to 400°F.
2. Cut off sides of eggplant circles to make square shapes. Place slices in a colander and toss with salt. Let sit 10 minutes, then rinse with water.
3. In a small bowl, add egg. In a second bowl, add almond meal and oregano, stirring well to combine. Dredge eggplant squares in egg, tap off any excess, and then dredge in almond meal. Place slices on one or two nonstick baking sheets.
4. Slowly drizzle olive oil to cover the top of each square. Bake 12 minutes.
5. Remove eggplant from oven and spoon marinara sauce onto the center of each square, leaving edges of eggplant uncovered. Sprinkle mozzarella on top of squares. Bake an additional 3 minutes until cheese has melted.

Per Serving: | Calories: 247 | Fat: 16.5g | Protein: 9.0g | Sodium: 322mg | Fiber: 9.3g | Carbohydrates: 19.5g | Net Carbohydrates: 10.2g | Sugar: 9.7g

Garlicky Parsnip and Carrot Fries

These Garlicky Parsnip and Carrot Fries are a great alternative to traditional potato fries. They're a little sweet and a little savory, full of micronutrients, and will keep you satisfied until your next meal.

* Under 500 Calories *

INGREDIENTS | SERVES 6

2 tablespoons garlic-infused olive oil

⅛ teaspoon wheat-free asafetida powder

2 teaspoons chopped fresh flat-leaf parsley

½ teaspoon sea salt

5 medium carrots, peeled and cut diagonally into 1"-thick slices

3 medium parsnips, peeled and cut diagonally into 1"-thick slices

1. Preheat oven to 400°F.
2. In a large bowl, combine oil, asafetida, parsley, and salt. Add carrots and parsnips to bowl and toss well to coat.
3. Place vegetables on a rimmed, ungreased baking sheet and roast 20 minutes, flipping pieces halfway through roasting. Parsnips and carrots should be crisp and golden brown.

Per Serving: | Calories: 94 | Fat: 4.5g | Protein: 1.0g | Sodium: 169mg | Fiber: 3.6g | Carbohydrates: 12.9g | Net Carbohydrates: 9.3g | Sugar: 4.5g

Quinoa Pizza Muffins

These Quinoa Pizza Muffins are a healthier, gluten-free twist on the classic fan favorite: English muffin pizzas. They'll satisfy your cravings for pizza with an added dose of nostalgia.

* Under 500 Calories *

INGREDIENTS | YIELDS 12 MUFFINS

1 cup uncooked quinoa, rinsed
2 cups water
2 large eggs, whisked
1½ cups shredded mozzarella cheese
½ cup chopped fresh spinach
¼ cup chopped fresh basil
1 teaspoon dried oregano
½ teaspoon salt
½ teaspoon freshly ground black pepper
1½ cups no-sugar-added marinara sauce

1. In a medium saucepan, combine quinoa with water. Bring to a boil over high heat. Reduce heat to low, cover, and simmer until quinoa is tender, about 15 minutes.
2. Preheat oven to 350°F. Grease a 12-cup muffin tin with cooking spray.
3. In saucepan, combine quinoa, eggs, cheese, spinach, basil, oregano, salt, and pepper.
4. Add ¼ cup mixture to each muffin well. Press down gently on mixture with back of a spoon or with your fingers.
5. Bake 20 minutes. Allow to cool 5 minutes and serve topped with marinara sauce.

Per Serving: 1 muffin | Calories: 119 | Fat: 4.4g | Protein: 6.7g | Sodium: 278mg | Fiber: 1.6g | Carbohydrates: 12.1g | Net Carbohydrates: 10.5g | Sugar: 1.7g

Raspberry Lemon Chia Seed Jam

This jam is delicious on a warm scone, on gluten-free toast with butter, or mixed into a tub of grass-fed or coconut-milk yogurt.

⋆ Under 500 Calories ⋆

INGREDIENTS | YIELDS 1 CUP

½ pint (6 ounces) fresh raspberries
1 tablespoon freshly squeezed lemon juice
1 tablespoon lemon zest
2½ tablespoons pure maple syrup
1 tablespoon chia seeds

1. Add fruit, lemon juice, lemon zest, and maple syrup to a small saucepan over medium-high heat. Cover. Stir occasionally until fruit begins to thicken, about 10 minutes.
2. Uncover and bring mixture to a boil over high heat (stirring often) until it reaches a saucelike consistency, about 5 minutes.
3. Stir in chia seeds and cook, uncovered, an additional 2 minutes. Stir and remove from heat.
4. Transfer jam to an airtight jar and refrigerate 3 hours before use. Jam will continue to thicken and can be refrigerated up to 2 weeks or frozen up to 2 months.

Per Serving: 2 tablespoons | Calories: 34 | Fat: 0.5g | Protein: 0.5g | Sodium: 1mg | Fiber: 1.9g | Carbohydrates: 7.5g | Net Carbohydrates: 5.6g | Sugar: 4.8g

Blueberry Chia Seed Jam

The chia seeds in this jam thicken it up so well that there's no need for pectin, an ingredient that you may not have on hand. The longer the jam sits in the refrigerator, the thicker it will become.

* Under 500 Calories *

INGREDIENTS | YIELDS 1 CUP

½ pint (6 ounces) fresh blueberries

1 tablespoon freshly squeezed lemon juice

2½ tablespoons pure maple syrup

1 tablespoon chia seeds

1. Add fruit, lemon juice, and maple syrup to a small saucepan over medium-high heat. Cover. Stir occasionally until fruit begins to thicken, about 10 minutes.
2. Uncover and bring mixture to a boil over high heat (stirring often) until it reaches a saucelike consistency, about 5 minutes.
3. Stir in chia seeds and cook, uncovered, an additional 2 minutes. Stir and remove from heat.
4. Transfer jam to an airtight jar and refrigerate 3 hours before use. Jam will continue to thicken and can be refrigerated up to 2 weeks or frozen up to 2 months.

Per Serving: 2 tablespoons | Calories: 34 | Fat: 0.4g | Protein: 0.4g | Sodium: 1mg | Fiber: 1.0g | Carbohydrates: 7.9g | Net Carbohydrates: 6.9g | Sugar: 5.9g

Chocolate Chip Energy Bites

These Chocolate Chip Energy Bites are the perfect snack-sized energy booster. Make a double batch and freeze some for later so you always have something quick and healthy to grab.

*** Under 500 Calories ***

INGREDIENTS | YIELDS 24 BITES

½ cup gluten-free oat bran
½ cup almond butter
⅓ cup pure maple syrup
1½ cups gluten-free quick-cooking oats
¼ cup pumpkin seeds
¼ cup dark chocolate chips
¼ cup no-sugar-added dried cranberries
¼ cup ground walnuts

1. Preheat oven to 375°F.
2. Add oat bran to an ungreased baking sheet and toast 7 minutes until lightly brown. Set aside.
3. Using a handheld or stand mixer, mix together almond butter and maple syrup on low speed until well combined.
4. Gradually add quick-cooking oats to butter mixture until combined, and then add pumpkin seeds, chocolate chips, cranberries, and walnuts. Mix until well combined.
5. Line a baking sheet with parchment paper.
6. Divide mixture into 24 even pieces. Gently roll each piece into a ball. Roll balls in toasted oat bran.
7. Refrigerate 2 hours to set or consume immediately. Can be stored in a freezer bag in the freezer up to 2 weeks.

Per Serving: 1 piece | Calories: 101 | Fat: 5.0g | Protein: 3.0g | Sodium: 1mg | Fiber: 2.0g | Carbohydrates: 11.1g | Net Carbohydrates: 9.1g | Sugar: 4.1g

Beet the Bloat

Beets are high in the vitamins, minerals, and antioxidants that promote your body's ability to function optimally. By combining beets with apples, lemon, ginger, and green tea, you can fuel your body with the nutrients it needs while optimizing its fat-burning potential.

* Under 500 Calories *

INGREDIENTS | SERVES 3

1 cup chopped beet greens
1 large beet, peeled and chopped
3 medium apples, peeled, cored, and chopped
½ medium lemon, peeled, white part removed
1 (¼") knob fresh ginger, peeled
2 cups green tea, divided

1. Add beet greens, beet, apples, lemon, ginger, and 1 cup tea to a blender and blend until thoroughly combined.
2. Add remaining 1 cup tea as needed while blending until desired consistency is achieved.

Per Serving: | Calories: 95 | Fat: 0.2g | Protein: 1.3g | Sodium: 49mg | Fiber: 3.6g | Carbohydrates: 25.1g | Net Carbohydrates: 21.5g | Sugar: 18.4g

Cleansing Cranberry Smoothie

If you're looking for a sweet and tangy treat, digestive relief, or both, this smoothie is for you. The combination of cranberries, cucumber, lemon, and ginger help cleanse your body and your palate.

* Under 500 Calories *

INGREDIENTS | SERVES 4

1 cup fresh watercress, thicker stems removed
2 pints fresh cranberries
2 medium cucumbers, peeled
½ medium lemon, peeled, white part removed
1 (½") knob fresh ginger, peeled
2 cups purified water, divided

1. Place watercress, cranberries, cucumbers, lemon, ginger, and 1 cup purified water in a blender and blend until thoroughly combined.
2. Add remaining 1 cup water as needed while blending until desired texture is achieved.

Per Serving: | Calories: 71 | Fat: 0.2g | Protein: 1.7g | Sodium: 8mg | Fiber: 5.6g | Carbohydrates: 18.5g | Net Carbohydrates: 12.9g | Sugar: 6.8g

The Cleansing Power of Cranberries

Cranberries are packed with powerful antioxidants and an abundance of vitamins, minerals, and phytochemicals. They help flush bad bacteria out of the urinary tract to promote bladder health and prevent infection.

Banana Coconut Bread

This delicious Banana Coconut Bread recipe can double as a dessert. Serve with fresh banana and strawberry slices for a complete, yummy treat.

* Under 500 Calories *

INGREDIENTS | SERVES 8

1¼ cups almond meal
2 teaspoons baking powder
¼ teaspoon baking soda
½ cup fruit purée of your choice (see sidebar)
¼ teaspoon ground cinnamon
2 large eggs
3 large ripe bananas, peeled and mashed
¼ cup flaxseed flour
½ cup chopped walnuts
1 cup shredded unsweetened coconut

Fruit Purées

Fruit purées are a great way to add sweetness to any recipe. Simply place your favorite fruit or fruits into a food processor and quickly pulse to a fine chop. Use in place of syrup or jam.

1. Preheat oven to 350°F. Grease a 9" × 5" loaf pan.
2. In a large bowl, mix together almond meal, baking powder, baking soda, fruit purée, cinnamon, eggs, bananas, and flaxseed flour.
3. Fold chopped walnuts and coconut into batter (do not overmix). Pour batter into prepared pan.
4. Bake 45 minutes until wooden toothpick comes out dry. Remove from heat.
5. Let bread sit 5 minutes, then transfer from pan to a wire rack and cool completely, about 1 hour.

Per Serving: | Calories: 302 | Fat: 21.6g | Protein: 8.4g | Sodium: 179mg | Fiber: 6.7g | Carbohydrate: 22.3g | Net Carbohydrates: 15.6g | Sugar: 9.2g

Turmeric-Spiced Kale Chips

These chips satisfy a craving for crunch without contributing any of the trans fats that come with deep-fried potato chips. Plus, the turmeric adds anti-inflammatory properties that, when combined with kale, make this snack quite the superfood.

* Under 500 Calories *

INGREDIENTS | SERVES 4

1 large bunch kale, washed and cut into ¾" pieces, stems and ribs removed
3 tablespoons olive oil
1 tablespoon ground turmeric
1 teaspoon sea salt

1. Preheat oven to 300°F.
2. In a medium bowl, mix kale, olive oil, turmeric, and salt, massaging it with your hands to fully incorporate.
3. Spread kale out on an ungreased baking sheet. Bake 10 minutes.
4. Flip kale over and bake another 10 minutes until chips are crunchy. Remove from oven and allow to cool 2 minutes before serving.

Per Serving: | Calories: 137 | Fat: 10.3g | Protein: 3.8g | Sodium: 422mg | Fiber: 3.6g | Carbohydrate: 8.9g | Net Carbohydrates: 5.3g | Sugar: 2.0g

Sardines in Red Pepper Cups

These cups can be put together in a few minutes and are ideal snacks for transporting. The sardines in this recipe are an often overlooked source of omega-3 fatty acids.

* Under 500 Calories *

INGREDIENTS | SERVES 1

1 medium red bell pepper, stemmed, halved, seeded, and ribs removed

1 (3.75-ounce) can no-salt-added, skinless, boneless sardines, drained

Juice of 1 medium lemon

¼ teaspoon freshly ground black pepper

Fill pepper halves with sardines. Sprinkle with lemon juice and pepper. Serve immediately.

Per Serving: | Calories: 160 | Fat: 6.0g | Protein: 15.3g | Sodium: 175mg | Fiber: 3.4g | Carbohydrate: 10.0g | Net Carbohydrates: 6.6g | Sugar: 5.7g

Broccoli, Pine Nut, and Apple Salad

This quick little salad will tide you over to your next meal. The broccoli and apple taste great together, and the toasted pine nuts add a little bit of crunch.

INGREDIENTS | SERVES 2

4 tablespoons extra-virgin olive oil
¾ cup pine nuts
2 cups fresh broccoli florets
2 cups cored and diced green apples
Juice of 1 medium lemon

1. Heat olive oil in a small frying pan 1 minute. Add pine nuts and sauté 3 minutes until golden brown.
2. In a medium bowl, mix broccoli and apples. Add pine nuts and toss.
3. Squeeze lemon juice over salad and serve.

Per Serving: | Calories: 675 | Fat: 55.6g | Protein: 10.0g | Sodium: 32mg | Fiber: 7.3g | Carbohydrate: 28.6g | Net Carbohydrates: 21.3g | Sugar: 14.2g

Roasted Spicy Pumpkin Seeds

Pumpkin seeds typically get thrown in the compost bin, but they're packed with nutrients, like manganese, magnesium, phosphorus, and iron. Instead of throwing pumpkin seeds away, try this easy recipe.

* Under 500 Calories *

INGREDIENTS | SERVES 6

3 cups raw pumpkin seeds
½ cup olive oil
½ teaspoon garlic powder
¼ teaspoon freshly ground black pepper

1. Preheat oven to 300°F.
2. In a medium bowl, mix together the pumpkin seeds, olive oil, garlic powder, and pepper until pumpkin seeds are evenly coated.
3. Spread seeds in an even layer on an ungreased baking sheet.
4. Bake 1 hour and 15 minutes, stirring every 15 minutes until toasted.

Per Serving: | Calories: 302 | Fat: 23.5g | Protein: 6.0g | Sodium: 6mg | Fiber: 5.9g | Carbohydrate: 17.5g | Net Carbohydrates: 11.6g | Sugar: 0.0g

Pumpkin Seed Benefits

Pumpkin seeds have great health benefits. They contain L-tryptophan, a compound found to naturally fight depression, and they are high in zinc, a mineral that protects against osteoporosis.

Stuffed Mushroom Caps

These appetizers are a bit more exciting than traditional bread crumb recipes. They are stuffed with protein and fats to ensure more macronutrients in each bite, and they're gluten-free!

* Under 500 Calories *

INGREDIENTS | SERVES 5

20 button mushrooms, stems removed and reserved

2 tablespoons avocado oil

½ pound 85 percent lean ground turkey, chopped

4 cloves garlic, peeled and minced

½ cup finely chopped walnuts

½ teaspoon freshly ground black pepper

1. Preheat oven to 350°F.
2. Hollow out mushroom caps. Place on a greased baking sheet. Dice mushroom stems and place in a medium bowl.
3. Heat avocado oil 1 minute in a medium frying pan. Add ground turkey and garlic and cook 8 minutes until turkey is no longer pink.
4. Add mushroom stems, nuts, and pepper to ground turkey and cook until mushrooms are soft, about 8 minutes.
5. Stuff turkey mixture into mushroom caps. Bake 20 minutes until golden brown on top.

Per Serving: | Calories: 262 | Fat: 19.7g | Protein: 15.6g | Sodium: 42mg | Fiber: 1.6g | Carbohydrate: 4.9g | Net Carbohydrates: 3.3g | Sugar: 1.8g

Tasty Baba Ghanoush

Eggplant is a great choice when looking for a healthy carbohydrate source. It has a slightly bitter taste, so be sure to cook it thoroughly.

* Under 500 Calories *

INGREDIENTS | SERVES 4

1 medium eggplant
2 tablespoons raw (nonroasted) tahini paste
¼ cup freshly squeezed lemon juice
4 cloves garlic, peeled
1 tablespoon olive oil

1. Preheat oven to 350°F.
2. Place eggplant on a greased baking sheet and bake 30 minutes, then let cool 25 minutes.
3. Cut eggplant into 1" squares.
4. Place eggplant along with remaining ingredients into food processor and pulse until smooth.
5. Refrigerate covered 30 minutes, then serve.

Per Serving: | Calories: 114 | Fat: 6.9g | Protein: 2.9g | Sodium: 8mg | Fiber: 4.9g | Carbohydrate: 12.1g | Net Carbohydrates: 7.2g | Sugar: 5.3g

Eggplant Benefits

Eggplant skin contains a potent antioxidant and free-radical scavenger called *nasunin*. This compound has been found to protect the fats that brain cells are composed of.

Paleo Chips

Give nacho chips a healthy makeover with this favorite that goes perfectly with guacamole and salsa.

* Under 500 Calories *

INGREDIENTS | SERVES 3

1 cup almond flour
½ cup flax meal
1 large egg
1 tablespoon peeled and minced garlic
1 tablespoon organic no-salt-added tomato paste
1 medium jalapeño pepper, stemmed, seeded, and chopped
1 teaspoon chili powder
½ teaspoon onion powder

1. Preheat oven to 350°F.
2. Combine all ingredients in food processor and blend completely.
3. Spread mixture evenly on a baking sheet covered with parchment paper. Bake 10 minutes.
4. Remove mixture from oven and cut into squares, then place back into oven and continue baking 10 minutes until crunchy.

Per Serving: | Calories: 344 | Fat: 26.3g | Protein: 14.7g | Sodium: 53mg | Fiber: 8.9g | Carbohydrate: 16.6g | Net Carbohydrates: 7.7g | Sugar: 2.4g

Complex Carbohydrates and the Paleolithic Diet

Looking to incorporate the Paleo Diet into your fast? The most difficult transition from a Neolithic diet to a Paleolithic diet is in the letting go of high-carbohydrate snack foods such as chips and pretzels. It can take a while to detox your body from these foods, especially if you're used to eating them regularly, but once you make the switch and stick with it, you won't look back.

Melon Salsa

This sweet Melon Salsa makes a great light snack paired with Paleo Chips (see recipe in this chapter). You can also use it as a topping on your favorite fish or poultry dishes.

* Under 500 Calories *

INGREDIENTS | SERVES 4

3 small beefsteak tomatoes, seeded and finely diced

½ medium honeydew melon, peeled, rind removed, and finely diced

1 medium cantaloupe, peeled, rind removed, and finely diced

1 cup peeled and minced red onion

½ medium jalapeño pepper, stemmed, seeded, and minced

½ cup chopped fresh cilantro

Juice of 1 large lime

1. In a large serving bowl, combine all ingredients and mix well.
2. Refrigerate covered 4 hours and serve.

Per Serving: | Calories: 121 | Fat: 0.4g | Protein: 3.0g | Sodium: 50mg | Fiber: 3.9g | Carbohydrate: 29.5g | Net Carbohydrates: 25.6g | Sugar: 24.6g

Melons

Melons are lower in sugar than other fruits, like pineapple and grapes. Cantaloupe and honeydew are great choices when you want to enjoy fruit but are trying to keep your sugar intake low.

Avocado Salad

This salad is light and refreshing, and the healthy fats in the avocado will help keep you full until your next meal, making it easier to stick to your fasting and feeding windows.

*** Under 500 Calories ***

INGREDIENTS | SERVES 4

2 ripe medium avocados, peeled, pitted, and diced

1 small sweet onion, peeled and chopped

1 medium red bell pepper, stemmed, seeded, and chopped

1 large vine-ripened tomato, chopped

¼ cup chopped fresh cilantro

Juice of ½ medium lime

1. In a medium bowl, combine all ingredients.
2. Refrigerate covered at least 2 hours before serving.

Per Serving: | Calories: 138 | Fat: 9.4g | Protein: 2.3g | Sodium: 9mg | Fiber: 6.1g | Carbohydrate: 11.4g | Net Carbohydrates: 5.3g | Sugar: 3.5g

Red Versus Green Peppers

Although green and red peppers are both healthy choices, red peppers contain a very high amount of vitamins A and C. One medium red pepper can contribute a whopping 75 percent of vitamin A and 253 percent of vitamin C, compared with 9 percent vitamin A and 159 percent vitamin C per medium green pepper.

Roasted Garlic and Red Pepper Hummus

This hummus recipe uses basic but flavor-packed ingredients that are usually already on hand. Pair with Paleo Chips (see recipe in this chapter) or vegetable sticks for a complete snack.

* Under 500 Calories *

INGREDIENTS | SERVES 8

2 cloves peeled and roasted garlic

2 cups canned (salt- and fat-free) garbanzo beans, drained

⅓ cup raw tahini

⅓ cup freshly squeezed lemon juice

½ cup chopped jarred roasted red peppers

¼ teaspoon dried basil

¼ teaspoon freshly ground black pepper

1. In a food processor, combine roasted garlic, garbanzo beans, tahini, lemon juice, roasted red peppers, and basil. Process until mixture is smooth.
2. Season with black pepper and transfer to a covered bowl to refrigerate until ready to serve.

Per Serving: | Calories: 116 | Fat: 5.6g | Protein: 5.0g | Sodium: 132mg | Fiber: 3.6g | Carbohydrates: 12.5g | Net Carbohydrates: 8.9g | Sugar: 0.8g

Spiced Mixed Nut Butter

Serve this nut butter with Paleo Chips (see recipe in this chapter), celery sticks, or plantain chips. You can even eat it right off the spoon for a quick, healthy dose of protein and fat. Refrigerate any leftovers.

⋆ Under 500 Calories ⋆

INGREDIENTS | SERVES 8

2 tablespoons sesame seeds

2 tablespoons ground dry-roasted unsalted almonds

2 tablespoons hulled sunflower seeds

½ tablespoon raw honey

¼ teaspoon ground cinnamon

⅛ teaspoon pumpkin pie spice

⅛ teaspoon unsweetened cocoa powder

1. Heat a large, deep nonstick sauté pan over medium heat 1 minute. Add sesame seeds, ground almonds, and sunflower seeds and toast 7 minutes until lightly browned, stirring frequently to prevent burning. Immediately transfer nuts to a bowl and let cool 5 minutes.
2. Combine cooled, toasted nuts along with the remaining ingredients in a blender or food processor and process until the desired consistency is reached, scraping down the sides of the jar or bowl as necessary. Refrigerate until ready to use.

Per Serving: | Calories: 42 | Fat: 3.3g | Protein: 1.2g | Sodium: 0mg | Fiber: 0.8g | Carbohydrates: 2.6g | Net Carbohydrates: 1.8g | Sugar: 1.2g

CHAPTER 11

Dessert

Baked Apples

These baked apples satisfy a sweet craving without any added sweeteners. Leave the skin on the apples for extra fiber.

* Under 500 Calories *

INGREDIENTS | SERVES 6

6 large Pink Lady apples, cores removed to ½" of bottom of apples

1 cup shredded unsweetened coconut

1 teaspoon ground cinnamon

1. Preheat oven to 350°F.
2. Place apples in a medium baking dish. Fill each apple center with coconut and sprinkle with cinnamon.
3. Bake 15 minutes. Apples are done when they are completely soft and brown on top.

Per Serving: | **Calories:** 203 | **Fat:** 8.0g | **Protein:** 1.4g | **Sodium:** 2mg | **Fiber:** 7.5g | **Carbohydrate:** 31.3g | **Net Carbohydrates:** 23.8g | **Sugar:** 21.6g

Cranberry Chutney

This Cranberry Chutney is a satisfying treat on its own, but it also makes a great topping for Chocolate Mug Cake or Banana Coconut "Nice" Cream (see both recipes in this chapter).

* Under 500 Calories *

INGREDIENTS | SERVES 2

2 cups fresh or frozen cranberries
¼ cup peeled and finely diced red onion
1 cup coconut sugar
6 whole cloves
¼ cup water

Combine all ingredients in a small, heavy-bottomed saucepot. Simmer on low heat 15 minutes until all cranberries are broken and have a saucy consistency. Remove from heat.

Per Serving: | Calories: 414 | Fat: 0.1g | Protein: 0.6g | Sodium: 2mg | Fiber: 4.9g | Carbohydrates: 110.1g | Net Carbohydrates: 105.2g | Sugar: 100.9g

Pink McIntosh Applesauce with Cranberry Chutney

Don't peel the apples before making this Pink McIntosh Applesauce. Cooking the apples with the skins on gives this sauce its distinctive pink color and provides extra nutrients.

* Under 500 Calories *

INGREDIENTS | SERVES 6

1 (2"-long) cinnamon stick

8 medium McIntosh plus 2 medium Red Delicious apples, cored and quartered

¼ cup coconut sugar

¼ cup water

Cranberry Chutney (see recipe in this chapter)

1. Warm cinnamon stick, dry, in a large, heavy-bottomed pot over medium-low heat 2 minutes. Reduce flame to low and add apples, sugar, and water. Cover tightly.
2. Simmer 40 minutes, then uncover and simmer an additional 10 minutes.
3. Strain sauce through a manual food mill or push it through a strainer with a flexible spatula.
4. Let cool 10 minutes and serve topped with a dollop of Cranberry Chutney.

Per Serving: | Calories: 340 | Fat: 0.0g | Protein: 1.0g | Sodium: 3mg | Fiber: 8.5g | Carbohydrates: 86.0g | Net Carbohydrates: 77.5g | Sugar: 72.8g

Chocolate Mug Cake

You can make this Chocolate Mug Cake lower in carbohydrates by replacing the maple syrup with stevia or monk fruit.

* Under 500 Calories *

INGREDIENTS | SERVES 1

¼ cup almond flour
1 tablespoon raw, unsweetened cacao powder
1½ tablespoons maple syrup
1 teaspoon unsweetened full-fat coconut milk
1 teaspoon coconut oil
1 teaspoon vanilla extract
1 large egg

1. Combine all ingredients in a large mug and whisk with a fork to combine.
2. Microwave 90 seconds until a toothpick inserted in center comes out clean.
3. Serve immediately.

Per Serving: | Calories: 388 | Fat: 24.0g | Protein: 13.4g | Sodium: 74mg | Fiber: 4.0g | Carbohydrates: 30.0g | Net Carbohydrates: 26.0g | Sugar: 19.9g

Raspberry Lemon Oatmeal Bars

These Raspberry Lemon Oatmeal Bars are sweet enough to satisfy a dessert craving but also healthy enough to eat for breakfast. Double the recipe and store some in the freezer. You can thaw them out and have a quick breakfast ready to go when it's time to break your fast.

* Under 500 Calories *

INGREDIENTS | SERVES 12

½ teaspoon coconut sugar
1¼ cups unsweetened almond milk
½ teaspoon alcohol-free vanilla extract
1 large egg
¼ cup pure maple syrup
3½ cups gluten-free quick-cooking oats
2 tablespoons freshly squeezed lemon juice
2 cups fresh raspberries

1. Preheat oven to 350°F.
2. In a large bowl, whisk together sugar, milk, vanilla, egg, and maple syrup. Add oats, lemon juice, and raspberries. Stir well to combine.
3. Pour mixture into a 9" × 13" greased baking dish and bake 25 minutes.
4. Allow to cool 1 hour, then cut into 12 small rectangles. Refrigerate in an airtight container until ready to serve.

Per Serving: | Calories: 143 | Fat: 2.5g | Protein: 5.0g | Sodium: 25mg | Fiber: 4.4g | Carbohydrates: 24.4g | Net Carbohydrates: 20.0g | Sugar: 5.8g

Peanut Butter Cookies

These cookies are very easy and quick to make and use minimal, natural ingredients. Make them in advance and store them for a quick dessert that you can eat before your feeding window ends.

* Under 500 Calories *

INGREDIENTS | YIELDS 18 COOKIES

1 cup all-natural no-sugar-added peanut butter
1 cup coconut sugar
1 teaspoon alcohol-free vanilla extract
1 tablespoon pure maple syrup
1 large egg
½ teaspoon sea salt

1. Preheat oven to 350°F.
2. In a medium bowl, mix together peanut butter, sugar, vanilla, maple syrup, and egg.
3. Spoon out 1 tablespoon dough for each cookie, form into a ball, and place about 1" apart on an ungreased baking sheet. Use prongs of a fork to gently press down and flatten cookies. Turn fork and press down again to make a crosshatch pattern. Lightly sprinkle salt on top of cookies.
4. Bake 5 minutes, then turn baking sheet 180 degrees and continue baking another 5 minutes. Cookies should be golden brown around the edges. Cool 10 minutes before serving.

Per Serving: 1 cookie | Calories: 136 | Fat: 7.8g | Protein: 3.9g | Sodium: 47mg | Fiber: 0.9g | Carbohydrates: 13.2g | Net Carbohydrates: 12.3g | Sugar: 11.8g

Peppermint Patties

These Peppermint Patties have all the flavor of the original without any of the artificial ingredients. You can freeze them and eat them right out of the freezer for a refreshing and delicious end-of-the-night treat.

* Under 500 Calories *

INGREDIENTS | YIELDS 24 PATTIES

2 cups shredded unsweetened coconut

¼ cup canned unsweetened full-fat coconut milk

¼ cup coconut oil

½ cup pure maple syrup

½ teaspoon alcohol-free peppermint extract

Water

2 cups dark chocolate chips

1. In a food processor, process coconut 30 seconds into a fine texture. Add milk, coconut oil, maple syrup, and peppermint extract to food processor and process 3 minutes to make a paste.
2. Shape paste into 1½" rounds, about ¼" thick, and place on a baking sheet covered with parchment paper. Place sheet in freezer 10 minutes.
3. To melt chocolate, place 1" water in a large skillet over medium heat. Place chocolate chips in a glass heatproof bowl and place bowl directly in water. Bring water to a simmer, then turn off heat and let chocolate sit until melted, about 5 minutes.
4. Remove patties from freezer. Place patties on tines of a fork and dip into melted chocolate until completely covered. Place patties back on parchment-lined baking sheet and return to freezer.
5. Allow chocolate shell to cool and harden about 30 minutes before serving. Store leftovers in an airtight container in refrigerator up to 2 weeks or in freezer up to 2 months.

Per Serving: 1 patty | Calories: 192 | Fat: 13.3g | Protein: 1.0g | Sodium: 1mg | Fiber: 2.7g | Carbohydrates: 16.9g | Net Carbohydrates: 14.2g | Sugar: 12.4g

Choose Your Chips

When choosing which kind of chocolate chips to use for a recipe, you have to consider your dietary needs. There are Paleo-approved chocolate chips and chips that are sweetened with stevia, so they fit well in a low-carbohydrate diet. There are also unsweetened chocolate chips that add a nice bitter complement to a sweet recipe. Avoid processed chips that use artificial ingredients like unnatural flavorings.

Paleo Fudge

This Paleo Fudge is not only Paleo, it's also gluten-free and low in FODMAPs. However, even if you're not following any of those dietary plans, you'll still swoon over its delicious chocolaty flavor.

* Under 500 Calories *

INGREDIENTS | YIELDS 10 PIECES

½ cup coconut oil
½ cup almond butter
½ cup unsweetened cocoa powder
¼ cup pure maple syrup
½ teaspoon alcohol-free vanilla extract

1. Heat coconut oil in microwave 45 seconds to melt. Blend with remaining ingredients in a food processor or blender until smooth, about 1 minute.
2. Place ten cupcake liners on an ungreased baking sheet or wide plate. Fill each cupcake liner ½" full with fudge mixture.
3. Refrigerate mixture 30 minutes or freeze 10 minutes. When firm, remove from the freezer.
4. Store fudge in between pieces of wax paper at room temperature in an airtight container up to 2 weeks or in refrigerator up to 3 weeks. You can also store in freezer up to 3 months, but to prevent ice crystals and freezer burn, store in bags within airtight container.

Per Serving: 1 piece | Calories: 201 | Fat: 17.1g | Protein: 3.5g | Sodium: 2mg | Fiber: 2.9g | Carbohydrates: 10.2g | Net Carbohydrates: 7.3g | Sugar: 5.4g

Maple Cinnamon Coconut Chia Seed Pudding

This Maple Cinnamon Coconut Chia Seed Pudding does double duty as a dessert and a breakfast. It can satisfy a sweet craving while also providing enough protein and healthy fat to keep you full until lunchtime.

* Under 500 Calories *

INGREDIENTS | SERVES 4

¼ cup chia seeds
1 cup unsweetened almond milk
2 tablespoons pure maple syrup
½ teaspoon alcohol-free vanilla extract
½ teaspoon ground cinnamon
2 tablespoons shredded unsweetened coconut
2 ripe medium bananas, peeled and sliced
20 medium fresh strawberries, hulled and chopped
¼ cup chopped walnuts

1. In a large bowl mix chia seeds, milk, maple syrup, vanilla, cinnamon, and coconut. Allow to sit 10 minutes and then stir every 15 minutes three times—an additional 45 minutes. Cover with plastic wrap and refrigerate overnight.
2. Layer bananas, pudding, and strawberries in four ice cream glasses, canning jars, or bowls. Top with walnuts and serve.

Per Serving: | Calories: 221 | Fat: 10.0g | Protein: 4.3g | Sodium: 48mg | Fiber: 7.7g | Carbohydrates: 31.6g | Net Carbohydrates: 23.9g | Sugar: 16.7g

Banana Coconut "Nice" Cream

Enjoy ice cream without the heavy cream, milk, or tablespoons of sugar—hence the "nice"!

* Under 500 Calories *

INGREDIENTS | SERVES 1

1 ripe medium banana, frozen with peel on

¼ teaspoon ground cinnamon

½ teaspoon shredded unsweetened coconut

1 tablespoon unsweetened almond milk

1. Remove peel from banana. Place banana and remaining ingredients in a blender or food processor and blend until smooth, about 1 minute.
2. Spoon mixture into a bowl and enjoy immediately!

Per Serving: | Calories: 112 | Fat: 0.9g | Protein: 1.4g | Sodium: 12mg | Fiber: 3.6g | Carbohydrates: 27.8g | Net Carbohydrates: 24.2g | Sugar: 14.5g

Mango Creamsicle Sorbet

When the weather is hot and you're looking for a cold, refreshing treat, try this homemade sorbet recipe.

* Under 500 Calories *

INGREDIENTS | SERVES 6

3 cups peeled and chopped fresh mangoes
½ cup cold water
1 cup shredded unsweetened coconut
2 tablespoons freshly squeezed lemon juice

1. In a food processor or blender, combine mangoes and water; cover and process 1 minute until smooth. Add coconut and lemon juice; cover and process another 1 minute until smooth.
2. Transfer mixture to covered container and freeze until solid, about 2 hours.

Per Serving: | Calories: 139 | Fat: 8.3g | Protein: 1.6g | Sodium: 0mg | Fiber: 4.0g | Carbohydrate: 16.3g | Net Carbohydrates: 12.3g | Sugar: 12.3g

Sorbet

Try this recipe with other favorite fruits. If the sorbet does not seem sweet enough, add honey to the next batch.

Rainbow Fruit Salad

You can't go wrong with this salad—it's juicy, fresh, naturally low in fat, and full of vitamins, minerals, and antioxidants. Enjoy it as a dessert or a side dish.

* Under 500 Calories *

INGREDIENTS | SERVES 12

1 large fresh mango, peeled and diced
2 cups fresh blueberries
1 cup peeled and sliced ripe bananas
2 cups hulled and halved fresh strawberries
2 cups seedless grapes
1 cup unpeeled and sliced nectarines
½ cup peeled and sliced kiwi fruit
⅓ cup freshly squeezed orange juice
2 tablespoons freshly squeezed lemon juice
1½ tablespoons raw honey
¼ teaspoon ground ginger
⅛ teaspoon ground nutmeg

1. In a large bowl, gently toss mangoes, blueberries, bananas, strawberries, grapes, nectarines, and kiwis together.
2. In a small bowl, mix orange juice, lemon juice, honey, ginger, and nutmeg together.
3. Refrigerate fruit covered until needed, up to 3 hours. Just before serving, pour honey-orange sauce over fruit and toss gently to coat.

Per Serving: | Calories: 88 | Fat: 0.3g | Protein: 1.2g | Sodium: 1mg | Fiber: 2.6g | Carbohydrate: 22.6g | Net Carbohydrates: 20.0g | Sugar: 17.4g

Banana Bread

This Banana Bread is a perfect dessert or breakfast treat. You can intensify the flavor by adding more ripe bananas.

*** Under 500 Calories ***

INGREDIENTS | SERVES 8

1¼ cups almond meal
2 teaspoons baking powder
¼ teaspoon baking soda
½ cup fruit purée of your choice (see sidebar in Chapter 10)
¼ teaspoon ground cinnamon
½ teaspoon alcohol-free vanilla extract
2 large eggs
3 large ripe bananas, peeled and mashed
¼ cup flaxseed flour
½ cup chopped walnuts
½ cup shredded unsweetened coconut

1. Preheat oven to 350°F. Spray a loaf pan with cooking spray.
2. In a large bowl, combine almond meal, baking powder, baking soda, fruit purée, cinnamon, and vanilla. Add eggs, bananas, and flaxseed flour and mix well.
3. Add walnuts and coconut and fold them into the batter.
4. Pour batter into loaf pan and bake 45 minutes.
5. Let cool in pan 5 minutes, then transfer to wire rack to cool completely, about 1 hour.

Per Serving: | Calories: 269 | Fat: 18.6g | Protein: 8.1g | Sodium: 179mg | Fiber: 5.7g | Carbohydrate: 21.0g | Net Carbohydrates: 15.3g | Sugar: 8.9g

A Note about Bananas

Bananas are highly nutritious, but when they're really ripe, all the starch they contain turns into sugar. If you have problems with insulin sensitivity or blood sugar regulation, it may be best to limit the number of bananas you eat.

Delicious Pumpkin Pudding

Pumpkin isn't just for the holidays! This pudding can satisfy a sweet craving at any time of the year and is jam-packed with vitamin A. Make sure you're using canned pumpkin and not pumpkin pie filling, which contains added sugar.

* Under 500 Calories *

INGREDIENTS | SERVES 8

2 large eggs
1 teaspoon ground cinnamon
½ teaspoon ground nutmeg
½ teaspoon ground cloves
½ teaspoon ground ginger
1 (15-ounce) can organic pumpkin
1 (13.5-ounce) can unsweetened full-fat coconut milk
½ cup crushed pecans

1. Preheat oven to 375°F. Grease an 8" × 8" square baking pan with cooking spray.
2. In a medium bowl, whisk eggs. Add spices and whisk again. Add pumpkin and milk to bowl and whisk thoroughly.
3. Pour batter into prepared pan, top with pecans, and bake 45 minutes. Remove from oven and allow to cool 15 minutes before serving.

Per Serving: | Calories: 179 | Fat: 15.5g | Protein: 3.8g | Sodium: 26mg | Fiber: 2.5g | Carbohydrate: 7.2g | Net Carbohydrates: 4.7g | Sugar: 2.1g

Heavenly Cookie Bars

These cookie bars are heavenly—and healthy! You'll enjoy the perfect pairing of the spices with raw honey, and your stomach will enjoy the natural ingredients.

* Under 500 Calories *

INGREDIENTS | YIELDS 48 BARS

2 cups raw honey
4 cups almond flour
½ teaspoon ground nutmeg
½ teaspoon ground ginger
½ cup chopped dried dates
2 cups ground walnuts
½ cup raisins

1. Preheat oven to 350°F. Line 2 baking sheets with parchment paper.
2. Warm honey in a small saucepan over low heat 2 minutes. Remove from heat and let cool slightly, about 2 minutes.
3. In a medium bowl, sift together flour and spices.
4. Add honey to flour mixture and stir until well blended. Stir in dates, walnuts, and raisins.
5. Use a roller to flatten dough to ¼" thickness and cut into 48 squares.
6. Place squares on prepared baking sheets and bake 10 minutes. Allow to cool 5 minutes before serving.

Per Serving: 1 bar | Calories: 127 | Fat: 6.8g | Protein: 2.6g | Sodium: 45g | Fiber: 1.5g | Carbohydrate: 16.6g | Net Carbohydrates: 15.1g | Sugar: 14.0g

Almond Butter Cookies

The only "sweetener" used in these Almond Butter Cookies is unsweetened applesauce, so they're a great low-sugar dessert that won't cause blood sugar and insulin spikes.

* Under 500 Calories *

INGREDIENTS | SERVES 12

1 cup almond butter
1 large egg white
2 tablespoons unsweetened applesauce
2 tablespoons shredded unsweetened coconut
1 tablespoon raw unsweetened cacao powder

1. Preheat oven to 375°F.
2. In a large bowl, beat all ingredients together to form a thick batter.
3. Place tablespoon-sized scoops of dough onto an ungreased baking sheet. Bake 12 minutes until cookies are lightly brown on top. Allow to cool 5 minutes before serving.

Per Serving: | Calories: 137 | Fat: 11.0g | Protein: 4.8g | Sodium: 5mg | Fiber: 2.4g | Carbohydrates: 4.7g | Net Carbohydrates: 2.3g | Sugar: 1.2g

Chocolate Coconut-Milk Cubes

These Chocolate Coconut-Milk Cubes are a great alternative to ice cream on a summer day—and can be a satisfying end to your feeding window. You can alter the flavor by changing the fruit purée that you add into the recipe.

⋆ Under 500 Calories ⋆

INGREDIENTS | SERVES 10

¾ cup raw unsweetened cacao powder

6 tablespoons fresh fruit purée of your choice (see sidebar in Chapter 10)

6 tablespoons coconut oil

6 tablespoons unsweetened full-fat coconut milk

3 tablespoons shredded unsweetened coconut

2 tablespoons raw cacao nibs

1 large ripe banana

1. In food processor, combine all ingredients and pulse until very smooth, about 2 minutes. Add water if the consistency is not fluid.
2. Pour mixture into ice cube trays or molds and freeze 2 hours before serving.

Per Serving: | Calories: 144 | Fat: 11.6g | Protein: 1.7g | Sodium: 2mg | Fiber: 2.5g | Carbohydrates: 8.7g | Net Carbohydrates: 6.2g | Sugar: 2.3g

Coconut

This recipe uses all the edible parts of the coconut—the meat, oil, and milk—making this dessert high in fiber and various vitamins and minerals. It's also high in medium-chain triglycerides (MCTs)—a specific kind of fat that can help control blood sugar, lower cholesterol, and contribute to weight loss. MCTs also help keep you full, so it will be easier to get through your fasting window.

Baked Bananas

This healthy dessert is sure to become a new favorite. You can even double the recipe and use it as a spread on your Flourless Banana Cinnamon Pancakes (see recipe in Chapter 7) or Banana Bread (see recipe in this chapter).

* Under 500 Calories *

INGREDIENTS | SERVES 4

4 small ripe bananas, peeled and cut lengthwise, then across into 8 slices

½ teaspoon grated orange rind

½ tablespoon fruit purée of your choice (see sidebar in Chapter 10)

1 tablespoon freshly squeezed lemon juice

⅛ teaspoon ground cinnamon

⅛ teaspoon ground nutmeg

1 tablespoon melted coconut oil

1 tablespoon raw cacao nibs

1. Preheat oven to 350°F.
2. Arrange banana slices in a small (8" × 8") greased baking pan.
3. Combine orange rind, fruit purée, lemon juice, cinnamon, nutmeg, and coconut oil and sprinkle evenly over bananas.
4. Bake uncovered 40 minutes, basting after 15 minutes with liquid in baking dish.
5. Sprinkle bananas with cacao nibs before serving.

Per Serving: | Calories: 130 | Fat: 4.1g | Protein: 1.2g | Sodium: 2mg | Fiber: 3.3g | Carbohydrate: 24.5g | Net Carbohydrates: 21.2g | Sugar: 12.7g

Strawberry Coconut Ice Cream

This Strawberry Coconut Ice Cream will satisfy your ice cream craving—without the dairy! Even if you do eat dairy, this decadent dessert will hit the spot.

* Under 500 Calories *

INGREDIENTS | SERVES 6

2 cups coconut cream
1¾ cups frozen sliced strawberries
¾ cup coconut sugar
2 teaspoons alcohol-free vanilla extract
¼ teaspoon salt

1. Purée together all ingredients until smooth and creamy, about 90 seconds.
2. Transfer mixture to a large freezer-proof baking or casserole dish and place uncovered in freezer.
3. Stir mixture every 30 minutes until a smooth ice cream forms, about 4 hours. If mixture gets too firm, transfer to a blender, process until smooth, then return to freezer.

Per Serving: | Calories: 373 | Fat: 26.1g | Protein: 3.1g | Sodium: 100mg | Fiber: 2.7g | Carbohydrates: 33.5g | Net Carbohydrates: 30.8g | Sugar: 26.2g

Easy Banana Date Cookies

The daily fast during Ramadan is traditionally broken with a date at sunset, and a version of these simple, refined-sugar–free cookies is popular in Islamic communities in North Africa.

* Under 500 Calories *

INGREDIENTS | YIELDS 12 COOKIES

1 cup chopped pitted dates
1 ripe medium banana, peeled
¼ teaspoon alcohol-free vanilla extract
1¾ cups shredded unsweetened coconut

1. Preheat oven to 375°F.
2. In a small bowl, cover dates in water and soak 10 minutes until softened. Drain.
3. In a food processor, blend dates, banana, and vanilla until almost smooth. Stir in coconut by hand until thick.
4. Drop generous tablespoonfuls of mixture onto a greased baking sheet. Bake 12 minutes. Remove from oven and allow to cool 10 minutes before serving. Cookies will be soft and chewy.

Per Serving: 1 cookie | Calories: 121 | Fat: 7.0g | Protein: 1.2g | Sodium: 0mg | Fiber: 3.6g | Carbohydrates: 14.6g | Net Carbohydrates: 11.0g | Sugar: 9.8g

Apricot Ginger Sorbet

This yummy sorbet is made with real fruit and contains no dairy, so it falls nicely into most eating plans.

* Under 500 Calories *

INGREDIENTS | SERVES 6

⅔ cup water

⅔ cup coconut sugar

2 teaspoons peeled and minced ginger

5 cups chopped apricots, fresh or frozen

3 tablespoons freshly squeezed lemon juice

1. In a small pot, bring water, sugar, and ginger to a boil over high heat. Reduce heat to low. Simmer 4 minutes until sugar is dissolved and a syrup forms. Allow to cool 10 minutes.
2. In a food processor or blender, purée sugar syrup, apricots, and lemon juice until smooth, about 2 minutes.
3. Transfer mixture to a large freezer-proof baking or casserole dish and place uncovered in freezer. Stir every 30 minutes until a smooth sorbet forms, about 4 hours. If mixture gets too firm, transfer to a blender, process until smooth, then return to freezer.

Per Serving: | Calories: 148 | Fat: 0.4g | Protein: 2.0g | Sodium: 1mg | Fiber: 2.8g | Carbohydrates: 37.3g | Net Carbohydrates: 34.5g | Sugar: 34.2g

Sugar-Free No-Bake Cocoa Balls

Craving a healthy chocolate snack? Try these fudgy little cocoa balls, similar to a soft, no-bake cookie but with no refined sugar.

* Under 500 Calories *

INGREDIENTS | SERVES 4

1 cup chopped pitted dates
1 cup walnuts
¼ cup unsweetened cocoa powder
1 tablespoon all-natural no-sugar-added peanut butter
¼ cup shredded unsweetened coconut

1. In a small bowl, cover dates in warm water and soak 10 minutes until softened. Drain.
2. In a food processor or blender, process dates, nuts, cocoa powder, and peanut butter until combined and sticky, about 3 minutes. Add coconut and process until coarse, about 1 minute.
3. Shape mixture into balls on a baking sheet and chill in refrigerator 1 hour.
4. If balls are too wet once chilled, add more nuts and coconut and reshape. If the balls are dry and crumbly, add just a touch of water and reshape. Enjoy!

Per Serving: | Calories: 337 | Fat: 21.4g | Protein: 7.1g | Sodium: 2mg | Fiber: 7.9g | Carbohydrates: 36.0g | Net Carbohydrates: 28.1g | Sugar: 24.5g

Variations

Roll these little balls in extra coconut shreds for a sweet presentation, or try them with carob powder instead of cocoa—they're just as satisfying. Don't have fresh dates on hand? Raisins may be substituted, but skip the soaking.

Apple Crumble

This crumble is a healthier twist on a traditional apple streusel recipe. The granola topping gives it that crunch of streusel but without any refined sugars or other undesirable ingredients.

INGREDIENTS | SERVES 2

2 tablespoons plus ¼ teaspoon coconut oil, divided

4 cups peeled, cored, and thinly sliced medium Granny Smith apples

¼ cup coconut sugar

1 tablespoon ground cinnamon

½ cup crushed raw almonds

½ cup Cinnamon Spice Granola (see recipe in Chapter 10)

1. Preheat oven to 375°F. Grease a 9" × 13" baking dish lightly with ¼ teaspoon coconut oil.
2. In a large mixing bowl, combine apple slices, coconut sugar, and cinnamon and toss to coat. Spread apples evenly in prepared baking dish.
3. In a medium mixing bowl, combine almonds, Cinnamon Spice Granola, and remaining coconut oil. Crumble mixture evenly over apples.
4. Bake 40 minutes until topping is golden brown. Remove from heat and allow to cool 20 minutes before serving.

Per Serving: | Calories: 941 | Fat: 65.8g | Protein: 8.0g | Sodium: 71mg | Fiber: 11.2g | Carbohydrates: 81.2g | Net Carbohydrates: 70.0g | Sugar: 55.5g

Fruit Salad with Ginger and Lemon Juice

Traditional fruit salad is a few fruits and melons thrown together and served. This recipe includes a tasty dressing of freshly squeezed lemon juice and minced ginger for a heightened flavor experience that will make fruit salad mean something completely new.

* Under 500 Calories *

INGREDIENTS | SERVES 2

1 grapefruit, peeled, seeded, and sectioned

1 cup pineapple chunks

1 cup green seedless grapes, sliced

1 medium Granny Smith apple, cored and chopped

1 cup peeled, seeded, and cubed cantaloupe

1 cup peeled, seeded, and cubed honeydew melon

3 tablespoons freshly squeezed lemon juice

2 tablespoons peeled and freshly grated ginger

½ cup shredded unsweetened coconut

¼ cup raw cacao nibs

1. In a mixing bowl, combine fruit, lemon juice, ginger, coconut, and cacao nibs. Toss to coat.
2. Divide salad between two salad bowls and serve.

Per Serving: | Calories: 459 | Fat: 17.9g | Protein: 5.0g | Sodium: 46mg | Fiber: 14.3g | Carbohydrates: 74.1g | Net Carbohydrates: 59.8g | Sugar: 44.5g

Citrus to Brighten Fruit Flavors

Most fruit salads are delicious just as they are, and it's pretty difficult to create a bad-tasting combination of sweet fruits. Even if you don't particularly like lemon juice or lime juice on its own, you may find that it is the perfect addition to your fruit salads because of its amazing ability to brighten the colors and the flavors of the fruit.

Sweet Potato Casserole with Walnut Topping

Carrot cake isn't the only way to serve vegetables as a dessert! This Sweet Potato Casserole with Walnut Topping is sweet, delicious, and loaded with vitamin A, which keeps your skin and your eyes healthy.

* Under 500 Calories *

INGREDIENTS | SERVES 10

Olive oil cooking spray
3 large sweet potatoes, peeled and cubed
1½ cups unsweetened vanilla almond milk
2 large eggs
1 teaspoon alcohol-free vanilla extract
1 teaspoon ground cinnamon
1 teaspoon ground cloves
½ cup coconut sugar, divided
1 teaspoon ground ginger
2 cups crushed walnuts
½ cup coconut oil

1. Preheat oven to 400°F. Grease a 9" × 13" baking dish with olive oil cooking spray.
2. In a large pot over medium heat, boil sweet potato cubes until soft, about 15 minutes.
3. Drain potatoes and mash completely in a large bowl. Add milk, eggs, vanilla, cinnamon, cloves, ¼ cup coconut sugar, and ginger to bowl and blend well.
4. Pour sweet potato mixture into prepared baking dish.
5. In a small bowl, combine walnuts, remaining ¼ cup coconut sugar, and coconut oil. Sprinkle walnut mixture over sweet potato mixture and bake 45 minutes until top is golden brown. Cool 10 minutes before serving.

Per Serving: | Calories: 302 | Fat: 21.6g | Protein: 4.7g | Sodium: 58mg | Fiber: 3.0g | Carbohydrates: 23.4g | Net Carbohydrates: 20.4g | Sugar: 13.7g

Maple Rice Pudding with Walnuts

This beautiful dish is not only packed with the amazing flavors of maple syrup and vanilla (and the added crunch of natural walnuts) but it's also free of refined sugars and loaded with compounds that protect your brain health.

* Under 500 Calories *

INGREDIENTS | SERVES 12

Olive oil cooking spray
3 cups uncooked brown rice
7 cups unsweetened vanilla almond milk
¼ cup coconut sugar
1 teaspoon alcohol-free vanilla extract
2 teaspoons ground cinnamon, divided
2 teaspoons ground nutmeg, divided
½ cup pure maple syrup
1 cup crushed walnuts

1. Preheat oven to 325°F. Grease a 9" × 13" casserole dish with olive oil cooking spray.
2. In a large mixing bowl, combine rice, milk, coconut sugar, vanilla, 1 teaspoon cinnamon, and 1 teaspoon nutmeg.
3. Pour mixture into prepared baking dish and drizzle with maple syrup. Sprinkle walnuts and remaining cinnamon and nutmeg evenly on top.
4. Bake 2 hours, stirring occasionally to fold in walnuts. Allow to cool 30 minutes before serving.

Per Serving: | Calories: 306 | Fat: 9.1g | Protein: 5.7g | Sodium: 108mg | Fiber: 3.2g | Carbohydrates: 52.1g | Net Carbohydrates: 48.9g | Sugar: 12.5g

Clean Dream Piecrust

Forget the store-bought piecrusts! This is a simple and quick no-bake piecrust that's crunchy and delicious. Use it for the pie recipes in this chapter—and any other pie you make from now on!

INGREDIENTS | YIELDS 1 PIECRUST

Olive oil cooking spray
4 cups macadamia nuts
1 cup coconut oil
5 dates, pitted

1. Grease a pie plate with olive oil cooking spray.
2. Combine all ingredients in a food processor and process until smooth.
3. Spoon mixture into greased pie pan and press to ¼" thickness. Refrigerate until ready to use.

Per Serving: ⅛ pie crust | Calories: 721 | Fat: 73.6g | Protein: 5.3g | Sodium: 2mg | Fiber: 5.6g | Carbohydrates: 12.2g | Net Carbohydrates: 6.6g | Sugar: 5.5g

Blueberry Pie

Scrumptious blueberry pie gets a healthy makeover in this recipe. Skip the sugar and let the sweetness of the blueberries speak for themselves!

INGREDIENTS | SERVES 8

3 dates, pitted

⅔ cup unsweetened full-fat coconut milk

3 cups fresh blueberries

1 prepared Clean Dream Piecrust (see recipe in this chapter)

1. In a blender, combine dates and milk until emulsified and thickened.
2. In a small pot over medium heat, bring milk and date mixture to a boil. Reduce heat to low, add blueberries, and simmer 5 minutes.
3. Remove blueberries from heat, and allow to cool 10 minutes.
4. Pour blueberries into prepared pie shell and refrigerate 5 hours or up to overnight before serving.

Per Serving: | Calories: 797 | Fat: 77.5g | Protein: 6.2g | Sodium: 4mg | Fiber: 7.1g | Carbohydrates: 22.8g | Net Carbohydrates: 15.7g | Sugar: 12.7g

Peach Tart

When peaches are in season, this scrumptious dessert is a must-make.

INGREDIENTS | SERVES 8

4 cups peeled and sliced fresh peaches

¼ cup coconut sugar

1 tablespoon freshly squeezed lemon juice

1 prepared Clean Dream Piecrust (see recipe in this chapter)

1. In a mixing bowl, combine peaches, coconut sugar, and lemon juice and toss to coat.
2. Pour peaches into prepared pie shell and refrigerate 5 hours or up to overnight before serving.

Per Serving: | Calories: 773 | Fat: 73.7g | Protein: 6.0g | Sodium: 2mg | Fiber: 6.8g | Carbohydrates: 25.7g | Net Carbohydrates: 18.9g | Sugar: 18.0g

Frozen: The Next Best Thing

If you're making a fruit recipe, you don't always have to wait until the fruit you crave is in season. Manufacturers have perfected the art of flash-freezing fruits at their peak to preserve the nutrients and vitamins.

Banana Sorbet

Ice cream and store-bought sorbets can be packed with sugar and impossible-to-pronounce ingredients. This recipe calls for only four ingredients and makes the perfect sweet treat.

⋆ Under 500 Calories ⋆

INGREDIENTS | SERVES 6

4 medium frozen whole bananas, peeled and bagged prior to freezing

2 teaspoons alcohol-free vanilla extract

1 teaspoon ground nutmeg

1 teaspoon pure maple syrup

1. In a blender, purée bananas and vanilla. While blending, add the nutmeg and maple syrup or honey.
2. Once fully puréed, pour banana mixture into six cups and freeze covered 10 minutes.
3. Serve with a spoon.

Per Serving: | Calories: 78 | Fat: 0.3g | Protein: 0.9g | Sodium: 0mg | Fiber: 2.1g | Carbohydrates: 19.1g | Net Carbohydrates: 17.0g | Sugar: 10.5g

Banana and Cacao Pudding

If you are craving chocolate, this healthy and creamy no-sugar-added recipe will hit the spot!

* Under 500 Calories *

INGREDIENTS | SERVES 2

3 large ripe bananas, peeled

1 tablespoon coconut oil

2 tablespoons raw unsweetened cacao powder

⅛ teaspoon salt

1. In a medium bowl, mash bananas with a potato masher. Add coconut oil and mash again to combine.
2. Add the cacao powder and mix well. Add salt and mix.
3. Enjoy as is, or use as a dip for apple wedges.

Per Serving: | Calories: 260 | Fat: 7.3g | Protein: 3.2g | Sodium: 147mg | Fiber: 6.3g | Carbohydrates: 49.6g | Net Carbohydrates: 43.3g | Sugar: 25.0g

APPENDIX A

Sample Two-Week Meal Plans

THE 16/8 METHOD					
Week One	*11 a.m.*	*1 p.m.*	*3 p.m.*	*5 p.m.*	*6:30 p.m.*
Monday	Autumn Breakfast Chia Bowl	Stuffed Eggs	Spicy Shrimp with Lemon Yogurt on Wilted Greens	Spinach and Feta–Stuffed Chicken Breasts	Sugar-Free No-Bake Cocoa Balls
Tuesday	Flourless Cinnamon Banana Pancakes	Salsa Fresca with plantain chips	Traditional Greek Salad	Lemon Thyme Chicken	Easy Banana Date Cookies
Wednesday	Chicken Sausage Patties and Vegetarian Hash	Cinnamon Spice Granola	Dandelion and White Bean Soup	Pork and Fennel Meatballs	Strawberry Coconut Ice Cream
Thursday	Overnight Almond Butter Pumpkin Spice Oats	Mini Baked Eggplant Pizza Bites	Wild Rice Salad with Mushrooms and Almonds	Stuffed Peppers with Ground Turkey	Chocolate Coconut-Milk Cubes
Friday	Huevos Rancheros Without Tortillas	Cranberry Almond Granola	Lentil Salad	Citrus Flank Steak	Almond Butter Cookies
Saturday	Gut-Friendly Smoothie	Garlicky Parsnip and Carrot Fries	Butter Lettuce Salad with Poached Eggs and Bacon	Chicken Burgers	Heavenly Cookie Bars
Sunday	Farmers' Scrambler	Chocolate Chip Energy Bites	Tarragon Lemon Chicken	Fish Curry	Delicious Pumpkin Pudding

THE 16/8 METHOD					
Week Two	*11 a.m.*	*1 p.m.*	*3 p.m.*	*5 p.m.*	*6:30 p.m.*
Monday	Very Vegetable Frittata	Beet the Bloat	Turkey Meatballs	Slow Cooker Chicken Tagine	Paleo Chocolate Bars
Tuesday	Pumpkin Spice Smoothie	Broccoli, Pine Nut, and Apple Salad	Coconut-Crumbed Chicken	Tuscan White Bean Soup	Banana Coconut "Nice" Cream
Wednesday	Bacon and Vegetable Omelet	Roasted Spicy Pumpkin Seeds	Paleo Stuffed Peppers	Vegan Chili	Maple Cinnamon Coconut Chia Seed Pudding
Thursday	Strawberry Banana Pancake	Stuffed Mushroom Caps	Chicken Soup with Asparagus	Eggplant Parmigiana	Paleo Fudge
Friday	Breakfast Salad	Spiced Mixed Nut Butter with celery or apple slices	Picadillo	Lentil-Stuffed Peppers	Peppermint Patties
Saturday	Raspberry Banana Mint Chia Pudding	Avocado Salad	Chickpeas in Potato Onion Curry	Marinated London Broil	Peanut Butter Cookies
Sunday	Pineapple Turmeric Smoothie	Blueberry Chia Seed Jam with gluten-free crackers	California Garden Salad with Avocado and Sprouts	Lamb Patties	Raspberry Lemon Oatmeal Bars

EAT STOP EAT					
Week One	*Breakfast*	*Snack*	*Lunch*	*Dinner*	*Dessert*
Monday	Autumn Breakfast Chia Bowl	Stuffed Eggs	Spicy Shrimp with Lemon Yogurt on Wilted Greens	Spinach and Feta–Stuffed Chicken Breasts	Sugar-Free No-Bake Cocoa Balls
Tuesday	Flourless Cinnamon Banana Pancakes	Salsa Fresca with plantain chips	Traditional Greek Salad	Lemon Thyme Chicken	Easy Banana Date Cookies
Wednesday	FAST				
Thursday	Overnight Almond Butter Pumpkin Spice Oats	Mini Baked Eggplant Pizza Bites	Wild Rice Salad with Mushrooms and Almonds	Stuffed Peppers with Ground Turkey	Chocolate Coconut-Milk Cubes
Friday	FAST				
Saturday	Gut-Friendly Smoothie	Garlicky Parsnip and Carrot Fries	Butter-Lettuce Salad with Poached Eggs and Bacon	Chicken Burgers	Heavenly Cookie Bars
Sunday	Farmers' Scrambler	Chocolate Chip Energy Bites	Tarragon Lemon Chicken	Fish Curry	Delicious Pumpkin Pudding

EAT STOP EAT					
Week Two	*Breakfast*	*Snack*	*Lunch*	*Dinner*	*Dessert*
Monday	Very Vegetable Frittata	Beet the Bloat	Turkey Meatballs	Slow Cooker Chicken Tagine	Paleo Chocolate Bars
Tuesday	Pumpkin Spice Smoothie	Broccoli, Pine Nut, and Apple Salad	Coconut-Crumbed Chicken	Tuscan White Bean Soup	Banana Coconut "Nice" Cream
Wednesday	FAST				
Thursday	Strawberry Banana Pancake	Stuffed Mushroom Caps	Chicken Soup with Asparagus	Eggplant Parmigiana	Paleo Fudge
Friday	FAST				
Saturday	Raspberry Banana Mint Chia Pudding	Avocado Salad	Chickpeas in Potato Onion Curry	Marinated London Broil	Peanut Butter Cookies
Sunday	Pineapple Turmeric Smoothie	Blueberry Chia Seed Jam with gluten-free crackers	California Garden Salad with Avocado and Sprouts	Lamb Patties	Raspberry Lemon Oatmeal Bars

THE 5:2 METHOD					
Week One	*Breakfast*	*Snack*	*Lunch*	*Dinner*	*Dessert*
Monday	Pumpkin Spice Smoothie	Sardines in Red Pepper Cups	Turkey Meatballs with Roasted Beet Slaw	Mediterranean Flaky Fish with Vegetables	Peppermint Patties
Tuesday	Roasted Vegetable Frittata	Broccoli, Pine Nut, and Apple Salad	Chicken Soup with Asparagus	Lentil-Stuffed Peppers	Blueberry Pie
Fasting Day	*Meal One*	*Meal Two*			
	Curried Shrimp with Vegetables	Pepper Steak			
	Breakfast	*Snack*	*Lunch*	*Dinner*	*Dessert*
Thursday	Salmon Omelet	Paleo Chips with Onion Jam	South American Chili	Beef with Spinach and Sweet Potatoes	Maple Rice Pudding with Walnuts
Fasting Day	*Meal One*	*Meal Two*			
	Pumpkin Maple Roast Chicken	Lentil-Stuffed Peppers			
	Breakfast	*Snack*	*Lunch*	*Dinner*	*Dessert*
Saturday	Bacon and Vegetable Omelet	Chocolate Chip Energy Bites	Tarragon Lemon Chicken	Zoodles with Pesto	Banana Sorbet
Sunday	Autumn Breakfast Chia Bowl	Chocolate Chip Energy Bites	Picadillo	Fish Curry	Baked Apples

THE 5:2 METHOD					
Week Two	*Breakfast*	*Snack*	*Lunch*	*Dinner*	*Dessert*
Monday	Very Vegetable Frittata	Mushroom-Stuffed Tomatoes	Traditional Greek Salad	Slow Cooker Chicken Tagine	Paleo Chocolate Bars
Tuesday	Raspberry Banana Mint Chia Pudding	Mini Baked Eggplant Pizza Bites	Dandelion and White Bean Soup	Stuffed Peppers with Ground Turkey	Rainbow Fruit Salad
Fasting Day	*Meal One*	*Meal Two*			
	Bacon and Vegetable Omelet	Vegan Chili			
	Breakfast	*Snack*	*Lunch*	*Dinner*	*Dessert*
Thursday	Farmers' Scrambler	Artichoke Dip with Paleo Chips	Coconut-Crumbed Chicken	Basic Baked Scallops	Peanut Butter Cookies
Fasting Day	*Meal One*	*Meal Two*			
	Chicken Sausage Patties and Vegetarian Hash	Coconut-Crumbed Chicken and Rutabaga Oven Fries			
	Breakfast	*Snack*	*Lunch*	*Dinner*	*Dessert*
Saturday	Overnight Almond Butter Pumpkin Spice Oats	Cleansing Cranberry Smoothie	Paleo Stuffed Peppers	Vegan Chili	Banana and Cacao Pudding
Sunday	Breakfast Casserole	Tasty Baba Ghanoush with Paleo Chips	Chickpeas in Potato Onion Curry	Smoky Black-Eyed Pea Soup with Sweet Potatoes and Mustard Greens	Raspberry Lemon Oatmeal Bars

ALTERNATE DAY FASTING					
Week One	*Breakfast*	*Snack*	*Lunch*	*Dinner*	*Dessert*
Monday	Autumn Breakfast Chia Bowl	Artichoke Dip with Paleo Chips	Spicy Shrimp with Lemon Yogurt on Wilted Greens	Spinach and Feta–Stuffed Chicken Breasts	Pink McIntosh Applesauce with Cranberry Chutney
Fasting Day	*Meal One*	*Meal Two*			
	Tomato Spinach Frittata Muffins	Lentil-Stuffed Peppers			
	Breakfast	*Snack*	*Lunch*	*Dinner*	*Dessert*
Wednesday	Flourless Banana Cinnamon Pancakes	Curry Dip with plantain chips	Wild Rice Salad with Mushrooms and Almonds	Pork and Fennel Meatballs	Paleo Fudge
Fasting Day	*Meal One*	*Meal Two*			
	Coconut Cacao Hazelnut Smoothie Bowl	Stuffed Peppers with Ground Turkey			
	Breakfast	*Snack*	*Lunch*	*Dinner*	*Dessert*
Friday	Overnight Almond Butter Pumpkin Spice Oats	Mushroom-Stuffed Tomatoes	Smooth Cauliflower Soup with Coriander	Salmon with Herbs	Maple Cinnamon Coconut Chia Seed Pudding
Fasting Day	*Meal One*	*Meal Two*			
	Mini Quiche	Chicken Burgers			
	Breakfast	*Snack*	*Lunch*	*Dinner*	*Dessert*
Sunday	Chicken Sausage Patties and Vegetarian Hash	Stuffed Eggs	Chicken Soup with Asparagus	Lentil Soup with Cumin	Delicious Pumpkin Pudding

ALTERNATE DAY FASTING					
Week Two					
Fasting Day	*Meal One*	*Meal Two*			
	Artichoke and Cheese Squares	Slow Cooker Chicken Tagine			
	Breakfast	*Snack*	*Lunch*	*Dinner*	*Dessert*
Tuesday	Roasted Vegetable Frittata	Mini Baked Eggplant Pizza Bites	Coconut-Crumbed Chicken	Zucchini "Lasagna"	Almond Butter Cookies
Fasting Day	*Meal One*	*Meal Two*			
	Tomato and Leek Frittata	Paleo Stuffed Peppers			
	Breakfast	*Snack*	*Lunch*	*Dinner*	*Dessert*
Thursday	Gut-Friendly Smoothie	Beet the Bloat	Pumpkin Soup with Caraway Seeds	Filet Mignon Salad	Apricot Ginger Sorbet
Fasting Day	*Meal One*	*Meal Two*			
	Bacon and Vegetable Omelet	Picadillo			
	Breakfast	*Snack*	*Lunch*	*Dinner*	*Dessert*
Saturday	Strawberry Banana Pancake	Avocado Salad	Chickpeas in Potato Onion Curry	Easy Pan Chicken	Fruit Salad with Ginger and Lemon Juice
Fasting Day	*Meal One*	*Meal Two*			
	Garlicky Vegetable-Packed Omelet	Lamb Patties			

APPENDIX B

Best Food Choices

Meat, Poultry, and Eggs

Choose organic whenever possible:

- Grass-fed beef
- Grass-fed lamb
- Pasture-raised pork
- Bison
- Venison
- Elk
- Pasture-raised chicken
- Pasture-raised duck
- Pasture-raised eggs

Seafood

- Wild-caught salmon
- Sardines
- Anchovies
- Herring
- Mackerel
- Clams
- Scallops
- Mussels
- Oysters
- Shrimp

Fruits and Vegetables

Choose organic whenever possible:

- Strawberries
- Spinach
- Nectarines
- Apples
- Grapes
- Peaches
- Cherries
- Pears
- Tomatoes
- Celery
- Potatoes
- Sweet bell peppers

The cleanest conventional produce:

- Avocados
- Sweet corn
- Pineapples
- Cabbages
- Onions
- Sweet peas (frozen)
- Papayas
- Asparagus
- Mangoes

- Eggplants
- Honeydew melons
- Kiwis
- Cantaloupes
- Cauliflower
- Broccoli

Grains and Legumes

- Brown rice
- Wild rice
- Amaranth
- Millet
- Teff
- Buckwheat
- Sorghum
- Quinoa
- Peas
- Black-eyed peas
- Lentils
- Black beans
- Garbanzo beans (chickpeas)
- Adzuki beans
- White beans
- Mung beans

Sweeteners

- Coconut sugar
- Date sugar
- Palm sugar
- Pure maple syrup
- Raw honey
- Molasses
- Monk fruit
- Stevia (sparingly)
- Erythritol (sparingly)

APPENDIX C

Recipes with Calorie Breakdown

Recipes under 100 Calories per Serving

Tomato Spinach Frittata Muffins
Calories: 69

Spicy Shrimp with Lemon Yogurt on Wilted Greens
Calories: 89

Roasted Beet Slaw
Calories: 91

Shredded Chicken Wraps
Calories: 68

Slow Cooker Mediterranean Stew
Calories: 82

Salsa Fresca (Pico de Gallo)
Calories: 15

Roasted Beets
Calories: 52

Raspberry Lemon Chia Seed Jam
Calories: 34

Blueberry Chia Seed Jam
Calories: 34

Garlicky Parsnip and Carrot Fries
Calories: 94

Spiced Mixed Nut Butter
Calories: 42

Rainbow Fruit Salad
Calories: 88

Banana Sorbet
Calories: 78

Onion Jam
Calories: 89

Beet the Bloat
Calories: 95

Cleansing Cranberry Smoothie
Calories: 71

Pork and Fennel Meatballs
Calories: 54

Recipes 100–250 Calories per Serving

Turkey, Egg White, and Hash Brown Bake
Calories: 137

South of the Border Scrambler
Calories: 239

Mini Quiche
Calories: 162

Farmers' Scrambler
Calories: 193

Vegetarian Hash
Calories: 119

Chicken Sausage Patties
Calories: 105

Pineapple Turmeric Smoothie
Calories: 226

Artichoke and Cheese Squares
Calories: 175

Roasted Vegetable Frittata
Calories: 233

Old-Fashioned Sweet Potato Hash Browns
Calories: 114

Heavenly Hash Browns
Calories: 120

Pumpkin Spice Smoothie
Calories: 150

Very Vegetable Frittata
Calories: 166

Carrot Thyme Soup
Calories: 204

Dandelion and White Bean Soup
Calories: 125

Wild Rice Salad with Mushrooms and Almonds
Calories: 216

Lentil Salad
Calories: 211

California Garden Salad with Avocado and Sprouts
Calories: 179

Pumpkin Soup with Caraway Seeds
Calories: 214

Smooth Cauliflower Soup with Coriander
Calories: 214

Vichyssoise (Potato and Leek Soup)
Calories: 101

Red Pepper Soup
Calories: 162

Curried Chicken Salad
Calories: 124

Chicken Soup with Asparagus
Calories: 190

Butter Lettuce Salad with Poached Eggs and Bacon
Calories: 198

Baked Meatballs
Calories: 171

Marinated London Broil
Calories: 170

Smoky Black-Eyed Pea Soup with Sweet Potatoes and Mustard Greens
Calories: 107

Lentil Soup with Cumin
Calories: 146

Tuscan White Bean Soup
Calories: 237

Chicken Burgers
Calories: 224

Mediterranean Flaky Fish with Vegetables
Calories: 230

Curry Dip
Calories: 174

Rutabaga Oven Fries
Calories: 102

Mushroom-Stuffed Tomatoes
Calories: 106

Stuffed Eggs
Calories: 161

Cranberry Almond Granola
Calories: 105

Mini Baked Eggplant Pizza Bites
Calories: 247

Quinoa Pizza Muffins
Calories: 119

Chocolate Chip Energy Bites
Calories: 101

Tasty Baba Ghanoush
Calories: 114

Melon Salsa
Calories: 121

Avocado Salad
Calories: 138

Roasted Garlic and Red Pepper Hummus
Calories: 116

Turmeric-Spiced Kale Chips
Calories: 137

Sardines in Red Pepper Cups
Calories: 160

Apricot Ginger Sorbet
Calories: 148

Baked Apples
Calories: 203

Raspberry Lemon Oatmeal Bars
Calories: 143

Peanut Butter Cookies
Calories: 136

Peppermint Patties
Calories: 192

Paleo Fudge
Calories: 201

Maple Cinnamon Coconut Chia Seed Pudding
Calories: 221

Banana Coconut "Nice" Cream
Calories: 112

Mango Creamsicle Sorbet
Calories: 139

Banana Bread
Calories: 269

Delicious Pumpkin Pudding
Calories: 179

Heavenly Cookie Bars
Calories: 127

Almond Butter Cookies
Calories: 137

Chocolate Coconut-Milk Cubes
Calories: 144

Baked Bananas
Calories: 130

Easy Banana Date Cookies
Calories: 121

Recipes 250–500 Calories per Serving

Autumn Breakfast Chia Bowl
Calories: 471

Cran-Orange Oatmeal
Calories: 487

Flourless Banana Cinnamon Pancakes
Calories: 262

Coconut Cacao Hazelnut Smoothie Bowl
Calories: 294

Overnight Almond Butter Pumpkin Spice Oats
Calories: 288

Spicy Kale Scramble
Calories: 359

Tomato and Leek Frittata
Calories: 258

Raspberry Banana Mint Chia Pudding
Calories: 313

Strawberry Banana Pancake
Calories: 272

Garlicky Vegetable-Packed Omelet
Calories: 254

Huevos Rancheros Without Tortillas
Calories: 289

Traditional Greek Salad
Calories: 253

Chicken Piccata
Calories: 295

Warm Spinach Salad with Potatoes, Red Onions, and Kalamata Olives
Calories: 269

Salmon Omelet
Calories: 484

Escarole with Rich Poultry Broth
Calories: 471

Chickpeas in Potato Onion Curry
Calories: 451

Chicken with Sautéed Tomatoes and Pine Nuts
Calories: 311

Zesty Pecan, Chicken, and Grape Salad
Calories: 279

Curried Shrimp with Vegetables
Calories: 310

Turkey Meatballs
Calories: 351

Coconut-Crumbed Chicken
Calories: 353

Paleo Stuffed Peppers
Calories: 397

South American Chili
Calories: 310

Tarragon Lemon Chicken
Calories: 255

Chicken Lettuce Cups
Calories: 305

Slow Cooker Chicken Tagine
Calories: 381

Zoodles with Pesto
Calories: 374

Citrus Flank Steak
Calories: 333

Vegan Chili
Calories: 263

Zucchini "Lasagna"
Calories: 341

Lamb Patties
Calories: 399

Lentil-Stuffed Peppers
Calories: 473

Lemon Thyme Chicken
Calories: 480

Spinach and Feta–Stuffed Chicken Breasts
Calories: 395

Salmon with Herbs
Calories: 342

Mushroom Pork Medallions
Calories: 311

Mexican-Style Chili
Calories: 401

Cinnamon Spice Granola
Calories: 387

Banana Coconut Bread
Calories: 302

Roasted Spicy Pumpkin Seeds
Calories: 302

Stuffed Mushroom Caps
Calories: 262

Paleo Chips
Calories: 344

Cranberry Chutney
Calories: 414

Pink McIntosh Applesauce with Cranberry Chutney
Calories: 340

Chocolate Mug Cake
Calories: 388

Strawberry Coconut Ice Cream
Calories: 373

Fruit Salad with Ginger and Lemon Juice
Calories: 459

Sweet Potato Casserole with Walnut Topping
Calories: 302

Maple Rice Pudding with Walnuts
Calories: 306

Sugar-Free No-Bake Cocoa Balls
Calories: 337

Banana and Cacao Pudding
Calories: 260

Recipes 500+ Calories per Serving

Breakfast Casserole
Calories: 581

Gut-Friendly Smoothie
Calories: 676

Breakfast Salad
Calories: 598

Bacon and Vegetable Omelet
Calories: 606

Picadillo
Calories: 538

Not Your Grandmother's Eggplant Parmigiana
Calories: 680

Fish Curry
Calories: 592

Filet Mignon Salad
Calories: 910

Stuffed Peppers with Ground Turkey
Calories: 779

Beef with Spinach and Sweet Potatoes
Calories: 779

Easy Pan Chicken
Calories: 663

Pumpkin Maple Roast Chicken
Calories: 526

Basic Baked Scallops
Calories: 540

Pepper Steak
Calories: 847

Artichoke Dip
Calories: 643

Broccoli, Pine Nut, and Apple Salad
Calories: 675

Apple Crumble
Calories: 941

Clean Dream Piecrust
Calories: 721

Blueberry Pie
Calories: 797

Peach Tart
Calories: 773

Standard US/Metric Measurement Conversions

VOLUME CONVERSIONS	
US Volume Measure	**Metric Equivalent**
⅛ teaspoon	0.5 milliliter
¼ teaspoon	1 milliliter
½ teaspoon	2 milliliters
1 teaspoon	5 milliliters
½ tablespoon	7 milliliters
1 tablespoon (3 teaspoons)	15 milliliters
2 tablespoons (1 fluid ounce)	30 milliliters
¼ cup (4 tablespoons)	60 milliliters
⅓ cup	80 milliliters
½ cup (4 fluid ounces)	125 milliliters
⅔ cup	160 milliliters
¾ cup (6 fluid ounces)	180 milliliters
1 cup (16 tablespoons)	250 milliliters
1 pint (2 cups)	500 milliliters
1 quart (4 cups)	1 liter (about)

WEIGHT CONVERSIONS	
US Weight Measure	**Metric Equivalent**
½ ounce	15 grams
1 ounce	30 grams
2 ounces	60 grams
3 ounces	85 grams
¼ pound (4 ounces)	115 grams
½ pound (8 ounces)	225 grams
¾ pound (12 ounces)	340 grams
1 pound (16 ounces)	454 grams

OVEN TEMPERATURE CONVERSIONS	
Degrees Fahrenheit	**Degrees Celsius**
200 degrees F	95 degrees C
250 degrees F	120 degrees C
275 degrees F	135 degrees C
300 degrees F	150 degrees C
325 degrees F	160 degrees C
350 degrees F	180 degrees C
375 degrees F	190 degrees C
400 degrees F	205 degrees C
425 degrees F	220 degrees C
450 degrees F	230 degrees C

BAKING PAN SIZES	
American	**Metric**
8 × 1½ inch round baking pan	20 × 4 cm cake tin
9 × 1½ inch round baking pan	23 × 3.5 cm cake tin
11 × 7 × 1½ inch baking pan	28 × 18 × 4 cm baking tin
13 × 9 × 2 inch baking pan	30 × 20 × 5 cm baking tin
2 quart rectangular baking dish	30 × 20 × 3 cm baking tin
15 × 10 × 2 inch baking pan	38 × 25 × 5 cm baking tin (Swiss roll tin)
9 inch pie plate	22 × 4 or 23 × 4 cm pie plate
7 or 8 inch springform pan	18 or 20 cm springform or loose bottom cake tin
9 × 5 × 3 inch loaf pan	23 × 13 × 7 cm or 2 lb narrow loaf or pâté tin
1½ quart casserole	1.5 liter casserole
2 quart casserole	2 liter casserole

Index

Note: Page numbers in **bold** indicate recipe lists of main categories.

About the Author

Lindsay Boyers, CHNC, is a holistic nutritionist with extensive experience in a wide range of dietary therapies. She also specializes in gut health, elimination diets, and identifying food sensitivities in her clients. Her articles on nutrition and health have been published on various health and wellness sites, including Healthline.com, Livestrong.com, and JillianMichaels.com. She is the author of *The Everything® Guide to Gut Health*, *The Everything® Metabolism Diet Cookbook*, *The Everything® Guide to the Ketogenic Diet*, *The Everything® Low-Carb Meal Prep Cookbook*, and *The Everything® Ketogenic Diet Cookbook*.